OVERKILL

HOW OUR NATION'S ABUSE OF ANTIBIOTICS AND OTHER GERM KILLERS IS HURTING YOUR HEALTH AND WHAT YOU CAN DO ABOUT IT

OVERKILL

DR. KIMBERLY M. THOMPSON
Harvard School of Public Health
with DEBRA FULGHUM BRUCE

FOREWORD BY GEORGE D. LUNDBERG, M.D.

Produced by The Philip Lief Group, Inc.

RODALE®

Notice
This book is intended as a reference volume only, not as a medical manual. The information given here is designed to help you make more informed decisions about your health. It is not intended as a substitute for any treatment that may have been prescribed by your doctor. If you suspect that you have a medical problem, seek competent medical help.

Printed in the United States of America

Rodale Inc. makes every effort to use acid-free ♾, recycled paper ♻.

Cover and interior designer: Christopher Rhoads

Library of Congress Cataloging-in-Publication Data
Thompson, Kimberly M.
Overkill : how our nation's abuse of antibiotics and other germ killers is hurting your health and what you can do about it / Kimberly M. Thompson, with Debra Fulghum Bruce ; foreword by George Lundberg.
p. cm.
Includes bibliographical references and index.
ISBN 1-57954-534-3 hardcover
1. Communicable diseases—Prevention. 2. Hygiene. 3. Drug resistance in microorganisms. 4. Antibiotics. I. Bruce, Debra Fulghum, date. II. Title.
RA643 .T48 2002
615'.329—dc21 2001007788

Distributed to the book trade by St. Martin's Press
2 4 6 8 10 9 7 5 3 1 hardcover

Visit us on the Web at www.rodalestore.com, or call us toll-free at (800) 848-4735.

RODALE
WE INSPIRE AND ENABLE PEOPLE TO IMPROVE THEIR LIVES AND THE WORLD AROUND THEM

To Kamran

ACKNOWLEDGMENTS

Any effort such as this one involves the help of many dedicated hands, gifted minds, and empathic hearts. I am indebted to the many family, friends, and colleagues who helped in the conception, writing, and production of this book. I thank Kamran, Deanna, Nima, Billie, and Kirk for their boundless support.

I thank my editors Judy Linden and Lynne Kirk at the Philip Lief Group for recognizing the timeliness of this book, for taking it from concept to reality, and for their nonstop enthusiasm and commitment.

I thank health journalist Debra Bruce for her experience and incredible ability to bring the scientific words together in a way that they can be easily understood, for many hours of research and phone calls, and for working with me with remarkable dedication to reach a clear final goal through the enormous stresses of meeting an aggressive deadline. Along with Debra, I thank her husband, Bob, for his support, patience, and advice, and her family, particularly her new granddaughter Zoe, for motivation and inspiration.

For his enthusiasm and eagerness to give his professional expertise, I thank Chris D. Meletis, N.D., dean of naturopathic medicine and chief medical officer at the National College of Naturopathic Medicine, for contributing the natural healing therapies given in chapters 3 and 4.

I similarly thank author and health columnist Laurel Vukovic for contributing the natural cleaners detailed in chapters 4 and 5.

I thank Drs. Harriet Burge, Skip Burkle, Donald Goldman, Harold Koenig, Joseph Li, George Lundberg, and Robert Tauxe for helpful comments that significantly improved the book. I particularly thank George Lundberg for his comments that led to the inclusion of substantive references and for writing an eloquent and compelling foreword.

I especially thank my editor at Rodale, Stephanie Tade, for her enthusiastic support throughout the publishing process. I thank Chris Potash and Jennifer Kushnier at Rodale for making everything fit and come together. For all of the many others at Rodale who have contributed to the making of this book in some way, thank you for believing in this project and helping to make *Overkill* a reality.

And finally I thank you, the reader, for going with me into the Age of Risk Management. With this book, I want to empower you to make better health choices about germs. I hope that this is the beginning of an ongoing adventure for all of us in changing the way we view our health risks from germs so that we can live active, purposeful lives.

CONTENTS

FOREWORD

The majority of us understand that most viral infections must run their course and that by using safe lifestyle approaches that are now standard in developed countries, most cases of parasitic disease can be prevented. But until very recently, most of us have erroneously adhered to the belief that the lethal threat of bacterial disease was a thing of the past, banished by antibiotics to the pages of old textbooks. We have known for at least 50 years about resistance to antibiotics, such that a prudent physician had to be sure to get antibiotic sensitivity tests on some organisms to guide antibiotic selection. But we had faith that when bacteria developed resistance to antibiotics, our fantastic pharmaceutical industry would simply make some new antibiotics—more expensive to be sure, with ever fancier names, and marketed aggressively, but effective nonetheless—bailing us out *ad infinitum*. Would that this could have been endlessly true.

In 1996, the *Journal of the American Medical Association* led a worldwide editorial effort, with 36 medical journals on every continent simultaneously dedicating many pages to the topic of emerging and reemerging microbial threats. This effort called widespread public and professional attention to the fact that we in medicine could no longer be deluded by the belief that the era of serious infectious disease was behind us. Two major events powered that conclusion and ignited a major effort to change the attitudes of doctors and patients alike: the HIV/AIDS epidemic and the increasing frequency of serious, even life-threatening, infections with bacteria dangerously resistant to antibiotics.

Attention was gained; attitudes began to shift; some good things happened. But for some people, the reaction became an overreaction, indeed almost a compulsion, to live germ-free. Some companies capitalized on this concern as an opportunity for marketing new germ-eradication products. We need to focus sensibly on the story of biology, that which narrates the cooperative or symbiotic, and the pathologic or beneficial relationships in this world.

Enter this book. A highly regarded expert on risk assessment, author Kimberly Thompson offers her unique perspectives on how to live sensibly in peace or war with our microbes. This book is a unique offering, tailored for the intelligent general reader who is interested in staying healthy and trying to keep his or her own family healthy without going overboard.

In life, everything has risk attached to it. This book demonstrates how the risks associated with germs can be understood and managed. Let it guide you to make intelligent choices. Read on, choose, and stay healthy.

George D. Lundberg, M.D.
Editor in Chief and Executive Vice President, Medscape
November 2001

INTRODUCTION

ARE THE GERMS WINNING?

It may seem surprising that germs are still a critical issue in the 21st century. After all, we're a technically sophisticated society with such health advancements as well-sealed clean homes, water disinfection, sterilization of medical equipment, refrigeration, indoor plumbing, immunizations, and antibiotics. All of these innovations have helped to control and eradicate infectious diseases and have improved the quality and length of our lives. For example, the average American baby born in 2000 is expected to live 80 years, compared to the 47 years expected for a baby born in 1900.

Nonetheless, at the beginning of a new millennium filled with medical promise and scientific breakthroughs, we face a public health crisis fueled by misinformation. The simple truth is this: Not only do we remain far from victory in the battle against infectious diseases, but overkill—our modern approach to germs that focuses on killing them beyond what is reasonable or necessary—often results in stronger strains of bacteria and more difficult-to-treat infections that can make the situation worse instead of better.

The tragic events of September 11, 2001, reminded all Americans of our vulnerability, both as a nation and as individuals. As a member of the National Academy of Sciences panel on arsenic in drinking water, I was briefing some staff members at the White House the morning of September 11. I can attest to my own fear as we ran from the building during the emergency evacuation just before American Airlines Flight 77 crashed into the Pentagon. The subsequent anthrax scares served as a dramatic warning that we must be better prepared as a nation for terrorist and biological attacks.

Perhaps what we haven't heard enough is that we must also prepare *as individuals*. This must start with a better public understanding about germ-related risks and what we can do to manage them—not just the bioterrorism risks, but the everyday risks too. Let's put this in perspective. People panicked when the first cases of anthrax were confirmed following the September 11 attacks, and yet at the same time, a study by researchers at the Centers for Disease Control and Prevention (CDC) in Atlanta had estimated that approximately 5,000 Americans die each year—more than 10 each day—as a result of food-borne illnesses.

In addition, our arsenal of pharmaceuticals is becoming less and less effective. The germs keep changing, becoming more resistant to the antibiotics and other antimicrobial agents that we rely on to kill them. A report from the Institute of Medicine estimated the annual cost of treating antibiotic-resistant infections could be as high as $30 billion. National and international agencies, including the U.S. Food and Drug Administration, the World Health Organization, the CDC, and popular books have sounded the alarm that the overuse and misuse of antibiotics is fueling a resistant-bacteria epidemic demonstrated by the following statistics and incidents:

- Thirty percent of the cases of *Streptococcus pneumoniae*, which causes meningitis, bloodstream infection, and pneumonia and is one of the most dangerous pathogens for children and the elderly, are now resistant to penicillin. Studies report outbreaks of resistant infections in day care centers.
- Gonorrhea infections resistant to penicillin and tetracycline became so widespread that the CDC recommended newly developed antibiotics like ciprofloxacin (Cipro) for treatment, and now reports of infections resistant to the antibiotics continue to emerge.
- A powerful, multidrug-resistant form of *Salmonella* has appeared in the United States, Canada, and Europe, in one case infecting farmers and their cattle.
- Several strains of *Staphylococcus aureus*, which causes the staph infections prevalent in hospitals, are now resistant to vancomycin, one of the most powerful antibiotics available.
- Strains of *Staphylococcus aureus* are now appearing outside of hospitals, with an outbreak involving seven members of a Vermont high school wrestling team in 1993 and 1994, documented in *Archives of Internal Medicine*.
- Tuberculosis is making a dramatic and frightening comeback, with cases on the rise, increasingly involving more of these resistant bacteria. For example, a study in the *Journal of Pediatrics* documented a 1993 outbreak of drug-resistant tuberculosis in a California high school.

Of course, many other examples exist. Even the reactions to the anthrax scares in October 2001 raised concern as millions of Americans rushed to get the antibiotic ciprofloxacin, also called Cipro, resulting in shortages of the drug in some pharmacies. Results of a study conducted late in 2001 suggested that approximately two million Americans might have actually taken Cipro unnecessarily, just as a precaution, thinking that they might have been eventually exposed to anthrax. We lack any information about how many of them may now harbor antibiotic-resistant bacteria as a result.

Public health agencies are so alarmed by the drastic increases in difficult-to-treat bacterial infections that they've mounted global campaigns to monitor them, and the medical establishment bombards physicians with data on the dangers of antibiotic overuse and misuse. Yet patients continue to clamor for the drugs. As pharmaceutical companies scramble to develop new prescription medicines to treat increasingly resistant strains of germs and manufacturers feed the public demand for nonprescription over-the-counter germ killers, the result is a marketplace crowded with a dizzying array of antimicrobial products. The problem is that no one is really talking to the public about its critical role in effective germ risk management. Unfortunately, hard evidence shows that if we don't stop the overkill as individuals, we not only risk sabotaging our own health, but we will inadvertently contribute to a serious public health crisis.

We've got to begin by educating ourselves about overkill. Even after all of the press coverage of anthrax contamination since September 11, 2001, confusion remains about what germs are, how they affect our health, and what we should do about them. Yet before we go further, check out the following myths about cleanliness and disease—along with some interesting scientific truths.

Myth: All bacteria are bad.

Truth: In large part, the impact of bacteria and viruses on your health depends on how and where they invade your body. Some "good" bacteria can be deadly if they get into the wrong place. For example, *Escherichia coli* (*E. coli*) live quite peacefully in your digestive tract, where they help you to process food; in fact, you depend on them for your survival. But if *E. coli* find their way into your bloodstream, they can be deadly. Even if a "bad" bacterium like *E. coli* O157:H7 makes it into your body, it can be harmless if it is cleared from your system without finding a way to attach to your body and reproduce.

Myth: Antibiotic overuse is not very common.

Truth: As early as 1998, a study by the Institute of Medicine estimated that approximately 20 to 50 percent of the 145 million annual antibiotic prescriptions given to outpatients and in emergency rooms, and 25 to 45 percent of the 190 million annual antibiotic prescriptions for hospitalized patients, are not medically justified. Antibiotics have no affect on nonbacterial illnesses, which include the flu, most colds, and some ear and sinus infections. Today's health professionals are in a very precarious position regarding antibiotic therapy, particularly if patients demand it—and studies show that many patients do. If a physician takes a wait-and-see approach, and the patient later develops a severe bacterial infection, that physician could be charged with negligence.

Myth: New medical breakthroughs are reducing the instance of asthma.

Truth: According to the National Heart, Lung, and Blood Institute, the incidence of asthma in the United States is now 1.75 times more common compared to what it was in 1980. Perhaps even more frightening, the incidence of asthma in children less than 4 years old is 2.6 times what it was in 1980. Although scientists are still exploring the relationships between immune development and disease, hygiene may play a vital role. Researchers have even developed one theory, called the Hygiene Hypothesis, that our modern, squeaky-clean lifestyles are partially to blame for a variety of illnesses, including allergies and asthma. Many other theories are also being investigated, including the possibility that children are spending more time in less clean environments and association of disease with the increase in smoking among women of childbearing age.

Myth: The bathroom is the most unsanitary room in the home.

Truth: Your kitchen has the highest levels of bacterial contamination, particularly in damp areas. Your sponge or dishcloth, drain, cutting board, and faucet handle are some of the biggest bacterial culprits in your home.

Myth: You can't do anything to protect yourself from germs—getting sick is normal.

Truth: A wide range of strategies exists to reduce the risks from germs; taking action is up to you. For people at very high risk, simple steps like boiling drinking water and eating only thoroughly cooked foods may dramatically reduce risks, but for most people this would be overkill. The action you take should be appropriate for your individual situation.

As a professional health-risk analyst, I have repeatedly raised the issue of germs as an urgent topic for public concern. Yet in addition to being a scientist, I'm a wife and the mother of two young children and like you, I worry about my family as I read the terrifying headlines—the ones that cover daily breaking news stories about the hazards of the germ world, whether it's *E. coli* on your toothbrush, *Salmonella* in your orange juice, or fears about anthrax. Instead of being scared by the news, however, I grow increasingly frustrated and disappointed because I realize that consumers aren't getting all the information they need to make informed decisions. Without that information, consumers may miss opportunities to avoid or prevent illness or worse in their family.

Most important to understand is that there is no one-size-fits-all approach when it comes to dealing responsibly with germs because it inevitably will go too far for some and not far enough for others. That's why I decided it was time to step in and apply my own particular expertise—assessing risks and identifying ways to reduce those risks—to balance the concerns of the medical and public health establishments with the needs of the average consumer. The cold, hard fact is that germs *do* cause illness. Yet many leading scientists are warning that we risk disaster if we continue to take antibiotics when they aren't needed, sterilize everything we touch, and attempt to shield our children from every germ.

So where should we draw the line? Again, a balanced approach is critical. And finding that proper balance—one that you tailor to your situation and that empowers you to play an active role in improving and protecting your health—is the purpose of this book.

How This Book Can Help

Unlike other books on the subject of germs and your health, *Overkill* places you, the reader, at center stage by focusing on your personal risk factors for contracting germ-related illnesses. As you read through the book, you will see that it quickly moves beyond a description of the bacterial problem and on to page after page of personalized self-help tips that you can use right now as you boost your immunity, stay healthy, and reduce your dependence on prescribed medications.

Here's how we'll accomplish this.

In chapter 1, Germs at a Glance, I'll give you the basic facts about germs—what they are, what they do, how they get around, and more. I also provide important historical context to explain how we got into the Age of Overkill and to help you appreciate the growing concern about antibiotic resistance. I share some eye-opening statistics to show you the global magnitude of this problem and to explain why it's time for all of us to enter the Age of Risk Management.

Chapter 2, Calculating Your Risk Quotient, is perhaps the most important chapter in the book. Here I'll help you focus on your personal health and that of your family using a detailed questionnaire that analyzes your risk factors for infection. Fifty questions are divided into five categories: Personal and Family Characteristics, Current

Health Status, Personal Hygiene and Home Care Practices, Food Preferences and Preparation, and Occupation and Leisure Activities. After you've completed this revealing questionnaire, you'll tally up your score to find your Risk Quotient (RQ), a number ranging from 1 (lowest risk) to 5 (highest risk). This number will be used throughout the remainder of the book to identify your optimal approach to health care, child care, home and work environments, and food preparation.

You'll learn how to improve your immunity and overall well-being in chapter 3, Protecting Your Health. Chris D. Meletis, N.D., author and dean of naturopathic medicine and chief medical officer at the National College of Naturopathic Medicine in Portland, Oregon, has provided us with a wide variety of natural remedies for the 31 conditions most commonly treated (or mistreated) with antibiotics, including acne, bronchitis, colds, ear infections, gum disease, sinus infections, and urinary tract infections. These remedies are custom-tailored for readers of every Risk Quotient. The goal of this chapter is to suggest some effective alternative ways to prevent and treat common conditions so that you don't call your doctor to demand a prescription for antibiotics every time you sneeze.

Chapter 4, Caring for Your Children, is a must-read for every parent or parent-to-be. Here I explain the Hygiene Hypothesis—the theory that a child's immune system requires stimulation to prevent an imbalance resulting in allergies, asthma, and even such autoimmune diseases as rheumatoid arthritis and diabetes—and other competing theories. Using the RQ calculated in chapter 2, you will learn how to determine the best day care center for your child, how often you should clean toys and playthings, and a variety of other tips designed to keep your child healthy. Natural remedies for 16 childhood conditions commonly treated with antibiotics are also included, along with warning signs that indicate your child requires immediate medical attention.

Household germs is a hot topic, with startling media stories about new strains of *E. coli* and other bacteria on everything from our cutting boards and sponges to toothbrushes and telephones. In chapter 5, Hygiene in the Home, I will accompany you on a virtual tour of your home and identify all the possible culprits lurking in your kitchen, bathroom, and laundry room as well as point out the "small stuff" that you don't have to worry about. As in the previous chapter, I will detail an individualized approach for handling hygiene based upon your Risk Quotient. I will also offer a variety of effective natural cleaners that can clean your home without setting up a breeding ground for resistant bacteria.

A CDC study estimates that food-borne microbes cause a staggering 76 million incidences of illness in the United States each year, resulting in more than 300,000 hospitalizations and approximately 5,000 deaths. In chapter 6, Eat, Drink, and Be . . . Wary? you'll learn how you and your family can avoid food-borne illness. I'll identify the steps you should take to store and prepare food in the safest way possible. In addition, I'll identify the most common food safety mistakes as well as offer simple solutions. I'll also give you the latest scoop on two controversial food issues: genetic engineering and irradiation.

I will go into more detail on how to provide additional safety and security for those at high risk or in special living circumstances in chapter 7, Strategies for Special Situations. Whether you're a 60-year-old grandparent about to spend a week caring for a new infant, a pregnant woman about to enter the hospital, a middle-aged person with a compromised immune system, or the child of an aging parent who is entering a nursing home, I will give suggestions on how you can optimize wellness in any situation.

And finally, in the Epilogue, I provide a look forward into the Age of Risk Management, particularly in these uncertain times when we continue to face the frightening threat of bioterrorism.

Here's to Your Health!

So, are the germs winning? Is cleanliness playing a dirty trick on us? No single easy answer applies to everyone. If we take the radical, dangerously obsessive approach toward germs that I call overkill, then the answer may well be yes. But it doesn't have to be that way. By learning more about germs, the risks they pose, and how we can reduce those risks, we can protect our own health and the health of the world at large. To that end, this book will provide you with the information and tools you need to determine a balanced approach that works for you and your family.

Let's get started!

1

GERMS AT A GLANCE

I have always been intrigued by the germ world and by the idea that something I couldn't see could make me sick. I first learned about germs when Mrs. Maffucci, my first grade teacher, discouraged the girls from "cootie kissing" by telling us "it spreads germs." That stopped us—for a while! At home, I heard more about germs from my parents, who were quite strict about cleanliness and hygiene and insisted that my brother and I wash our hands to "kill the germs" before eating.

But it wasn't until high school biology class that my concept of germs was first challenged. As I peered through a microscope in the lab, an incredible new world opened up to me. I saw magnified cell parts, constantly in motion, dividing and multiplying. I learned that while some bacteria can hurt us, others actually *help* us. The realization that life existed on such a small scale was incredibly awesome.

To teach us how quickly bacteria can multiply, one of my high school teachers used an ingenious technique. He posed the following question: "Would you rather have $100 a day for 30 days, or put a penny into a bank where your money would double every day for 30 days?" He grinned as most students quickly chose the first option—after all, not many high school students will pass up $100 for a penny! But I realized that while $100 a day for 30 days would yield $3,000, the doubled return from a single cent would grow to over $5 million in the course of a month. (If you don't believe it, get out a calculator and see for yourself!) I recalled this ingenious teaching technique when I later read Michael Crichton's best-selling novel *The Andromeda Strain*, which describes in terrifying detail how a single *E. coli* bacterium could grow into a "super-colony" equal in size and weight to the entire planet Earth—in just 1 day.

Several inspirational college professors continued to fuel my interest in science, but germs never impressed me as a major personal or public health risk. Just like all college students, I had occasional bouts of upset stomach or strep throat, but I was fortunate enough to live in the miraculous age of modern medicine. I took it for granted that immunization and antibiotics would act like a suit of armor, protecting me from germs. If I got sick, it didn't worry me—it was just an inconvenience that forced me to visit the doctor for more miracle drugs.

Then, about 5 years ago, my viewpoint began changing. During a luncheon in Washington, D.C., I sat next to one of the keynote speakers. The waiters served us the same meal, and when our iced teas arrived, I noticed that they were cloudy. I hesitantly took a sip of mine, but noting that it tasted sour, I left the rest untouched. The speaker took a sip of his tea, added more sugar, and drank the entire glass and most of a second one. I learned the next day that his talk was canceled because he was too sick to leave his room. This made me pay a lot more attention to the food I ate both at home and while dining out. It also illustrated the danger of bacteria in food as I listened to presentations about assessments of food-borne risks made by speakers from the U. S. Food and Drug Administration (FDA).

Around the same time, I also began to hear about increasing difficulties in treating drug-resistant cases of tuberculosis and other diseases, especially those that are prevalent in hospital settings. I was surprised to learn that many of these difficult-to-treat infections result from our overuse and misuse of antibiotics. The idea that antibiotics—the most powerful weapons in our germ-fighting arsenal—were becoming less effective made me realize that the Age of Miracles could soon give way to a new age.

Then one morning I came in to work and heard that a colleague and his wife had lost their baby daughter suddenly to the bacterial disease meningitis after returning from a vacation. Everyone was stunned by the news. At that sad moment, I appreciated that even today, germs still can kill and devastate people's lives, and I recognized that in my research on children's health risks I could not count germs out. As I drove home that day, I thought about how germs can hurt us when we least expect it, endangering those sitting right near us—or those most precious to us—and I appreciated that the human struggle with infectious diseases was far from over.

Since then, germ risks have occupied part of my research. In 2000, I was delighted that the FDA asked me to comment on its proposed decision-making strategy regarding the use of antibiotics in livestock. For many years, farmers have given these drugs to cows, pigs, and poultry, not only to combat disease but also to encourage growth in healthy animals. Some estimates suggest that more than half of all antibiotics used in the nation are used on livestock. Although this practice may help to keep harmful bacteria out of our food, it may also produce strains of bacteria that are resistant to drugs and that might be passed along to the people eating this food.

During these hearings, I was privileged to meet with distinguished experts and hear a variety of opinions on the issue, but remarkably, everyone agreed that members of the public need to know more about the nature of germs. Several participants at the FDA meeting suggested that, with my strong background in risk analysis, I could act as a voice of reason and separate the facts from the hype, helping consumers to understand their individual risks and avoid overkill. That meeting and my ride on the Washington, D.C., Metro back to the airport with several speakers provided the motivation I needed to write this book.

Defining "Germs"

Most people use the words *germs* and *bacteria* interchangeably, and I generally do the same throughout this book. Technically, germs are defined as any microorganisms or microbes—tiny bits of life too small to see without a microscope—that may cause disease, including bacteria and viruses. You may have noticed that the examples so far have mainly involved bacteria. This book concentrates on bacteria because most of our germ-killing actions focus on them, and their increasing resistance to antibiotics poses a grave risk to public health.

Before we go on, let's distinguish bacteria from other disease-causing organisms.

Bacteria (plural of *bacterium*). Simple, single-celled organisms without a defined nucleus. They come in different shapes: spherical (coccus), rodlike (bacillus), or spiral (spirochete). Fossil records suggest the presence of bacteria on Earth several billions of years ago, and bacteria were essentially the only life forms on the planet until a little more

What's in a Name?

Like all life forms, bacteria are identified with scientific names like *Escherichia coli* and *Lactobacillus acidophilus*. The first name signifies the genus, or type, and the second name indicates the unique species. The first name is often abbreviated to a capital letter followed by a period, so you'll see bacterial nicknames like *E. coli* or *L. acidophilus*. They mean the same thing as the full name; they're just simpler to use.

Bacteria can also be categorized into subtypes, or strains. For example, in the introduction I made mention of the highly dangerous *E. coli* O157:H7.

than 500 million years ago. Scientifically speaking, the rest of us are new kids on the block in comparison. Bacteria live everywhere on Earth, abound on almost every known surface, and they possess the ability to adapt to a wide variety of environmental circumstances. Consequently, scientists constantly discover new species, and some estimate that while only a few thousand species have been named and identified, there may be millions of species of bacteria. The great majority of these species are harmless to humans; in fact, our lives depend on some of them, like the bacteria that live in our intestines and aid in our digestion, those that break down dead organic matter or convert nitrogen into usable form in soil for plants, and the ones we use extensively in the treatment of sewage. And yet, as we have seen already, some bacteria can kill.

Fungi (plural of *fungus*). Single-celled microorganisms that differ from bacteria in that they have defined nuclei. The world of fungi includes yeasts, molds, mildews, rusts, and mushrooms.

Viruses (plural of *virus*). Fragments of genetic material that depend on other cells for their survival. Viruses invade the host cell and insert their genetic material into the host's genetic code, making the cell unable to reproduce, killing it, or turning it into a kind of machine that makes copies of the virus. Viruses are responsible for many serious diseases like AIDS and some forms of hepatitis, as well as most colds, the flu, and warts.

Parasites (plural of *parasite*). Organisms that live dependently in or on another organism and move from host to host. Lice are an example—they live on the scalp of a host and can be transmitted to others.

Our remarkable discoveries about disease-causing organisms over the last few decades have enabled us to develop a vast array of products to wipe out each type: antibiotics and antibacterials to kill bacteria, antifungal agents to kill fungi, antiviral agents to kill viruses, and antiparasitic products to kill parasites. It's important to understand that products designed to destroy one type of organism usually don't work on another type—and can even encourage the rapid growth of another type. This is why it's so important to understand the differences among disease-causing organisms and how they function.

10 Bacterial Basics

Fact 1: Bacteria can grow very quickly.

As I learned in high school, most bacteria grow by dividing in half, forming two cells from one. If left unchecked, this process can result in millions of cells from a single cell. This is why we may become suddenly and seriously ill from bacterial infections. If you've ever had food poisoning—and it's a good bet that you have at least once in your life—then you're familiar with the fact that germs can make you very sick very quickly.

Fact 2: Bacteria compete with other organisms.

The fact that bacteria grow and reproduce so quickly might lead you to wonder why they haven't taken over the world. Like all living organisms, germs require a supportive environment, with food to fuel them, a comfortable temperature range to grow in, and the means to dispose of wastes so they don't poison themselves. Other microorganisms (such as fungi and parasites) and macroorganisms (such as plants, animals, and people) compete with bacteria for these resources, and competition keeps the numbers of bacteria in check.

Fact 3: Some germs live cooperatively with other organisms.

One organism's waste matter can provide the sustenance for another organism to flourish. For example, *E. coli* inhabit the intestines of human beings and help us to digest food. This environment would prove hostile to most creatures, but fortunately for us, *E. coli* thrive.

Fact 4: The same germ can be harmless to one species and lethal to another.

For example, *E. coli* O157:H7 (a deadly strain that is quite different from the benign *E. coli* mentioned above) and *Salmonella typhi* are harmless to cows and chickens, respectively, but can cause bloody diarrhea and sometimes death in humans. On the other hand, *Actinobacillus pleuropneumoniae*, which causes respiratory disease in pigs, resulting in devastating economic losses to farmers, does not affect people.

Fact 5: Your body is a harsh environment for bacteria.

While there are some notable exceptions, your body generally is not a hospitable place for harmful germs, and only small numbers are able to survive and reproduce—usually not enough to cause disease. While bacteria tend to "stick together," forming colonies and clustering together for defense, it often takes thousands, even millions of bacteria to result in symptoms, and your whole body works hard to ensure that doesn't happen.

Your natural defense mechanisms include your skin, which forms a protective barrier against the outside world; secretions like tears, sweat, and stomach acid, which trap and destroy invaders; and bodily processes like sneezing, coughing, diarrhea, and vomiting, which can quickly remove foreign matter from your body. If invaders make it past the front-line defenses, they face an even more powerful force: your immune system. Its workings are so complex and amazing that an entire chapter or book could be devoted to it. For our purposes, however, it's enough to know that your immune system includes the thymus gland, tonsils, spleen, and a system of lymphatic vessels similar to your circulatory system that transport a clear fluid called lymph throughout your body, with periodic stops at lima bean-shaped structures called lymph nodes, where invaders are filtered out and destroyed.

Fact 6: Bacteria enter our bodies in several ways.

Germs are truly everywhere—they exist on all surfaces, including every inch of our bodies. So it's not surprising that they can enter our bodies in a number of ways:

- Inhalation—breathing in germs through the nose or mouth, such as when someone with a respiratory infection sneezes or coughs near you
- Ingestion—eating food or drinking liquid that contains harmful bacteria, such as those left out of the refrigerator for too long
- Contact—transferred by touching the skin, eyes, nose, or mouth, such as by a kiss from a sniffling loved one

• Sex—transmission through a reproductive organ, either through sex, childbirth, or via infection associated with birth control devices or tampons

• Injection—passed by a bite from an infected animal or insect, or through a puncture by a needle or some other unsterilized sharp object

Fact 7: Sometimes the bacteria themselves don't cause the illness; other times they do.

In some cases, the illness results from the toxins released by the bacteria. For example, botulism is caused by a potent toxin produced by the bacterium *Clostridium botulinum*, tetanus (or lockjaw) by a toxin produced by *Clostridium tetani*, and diphtheria by the toxin formed by *Corynebacterium diphtheriae*. Other illnesses are caused by the presence of the bacteria themselves, like toxic shock syndrome from *Staphylococcus aureus* and diarrhea from different species of *Campylobacter*.

Fact 8: Bacteria can evolve quickly in response to their environments.

Bacteria can change their genetic makeup each time they divide. Since division can occur as often as every 20 minutes, bacteria adapt to their surroundings very quickly. This is one of the reasons they've survived longer than all other creatures—and why they've become resistant to so many drugs used to kill them. You'll read more about this later in this chapter.

Fact 9: We do not know everything about germs.

Each day we're finding new germs and learning new things about the germs we already know about. Uncertainty is expected because bacteria are constantly changing. Thus, while our ability to diagnose and treat infections continues to improve, new strains of germs continue to challenge us. As noted in a study by researchers at the Centers for Disease Control and Prevention (CDC) in Atlanta, even 20 years ago we did not recognize many of the pathogens that cause food-borne illness.

Fact 10: People respond differently to germs.

Remarkably, some people exposed to a disease-causing germ can experience no symptoms, while others exposed to the same germ might end up in the hospital. These different reactions may be related to genetic makeup or due to general health and environmental conditions or combinations of these. Again, this means that a one-size-fits-all solution won't work. Not only is your situation different from that faced by others, but also it may be different today from what it was several years ago for you.

Germs through the Ages

Now that you've learned the key facts about bacteria and the other kinds of germs, let's look back to see how we arrived at our current crisis situation. Our story begins with humans living in the Age of Ignorance, where we struggled with infectious diseases, attributing them to evil spirits or the wrath of God. Scientific observation led to an Age of Discovery, where increased understanding of how germs work empowered us to kill and control them. This led to an Age of Miracles, with new drugs saving untold millions of lives, giving way to the current Age of Overkill, when bacteria have learned to outsmart our drugs.

Through the ages, thousands of scientists have made vital contributions to our current knowledge about bacteria, but here I'll simply touch upon a few select pioneers to provide a small sense of the amazing progress that has occurred.

Some Heroes of Germ History

1683: Antonie van Leeuwenhoek, using his perfected microscope, discovers bacteria.
1721: Cotton Mather designs an experiment showing the benefits of smallpox variolation.
1796: Edward Jenner develops the first smallpox vaccine.
1847: Ignaz Semmelweis demonstrates that hand washing prevents the spread of childbed fever.
1854: John Snow conducts studies on cholera and the water supply.
1867: Joseph Lister practices antiseptic surgery.
1876: Robert Koch establishes scientific rules for linking bacteria to disease.
1881: Louis Pasteur demonstrates anthrax vaccination on farm animals.
1928: Alexander Fleming discovers penicillin.
1935: Howard Florey begins testing penicillin at Oxford University.

The Age of Ignorance

Before we discovered germs and learned how to control them, life expectancy was incredibly low. While some well-known historical figures lived long lives—including Sophocles (who died at 90), Michelangelo, Sir Isaac Newton, Voltaire, and Benjamin Franklin (all of whom died in their 80s)—most people born before 1900 could expect to live on average around 40 years, and many children died before puberty. Infectious diseases played a major role in the annual death toll, with malaria, smallpox, measles, and gonorrhea devastating many early civilizations. When a fast-killing disease called the Black Plague, caused by the bacterium *Yersinia pestis*, swept through Europe in the 14th century, it wiped out more than a third of the entire population. Previously, plague in the 5th century contributed significantly to the fall of the Roman Empire, helping to plunge human civilization into the Dark Ages.

Given the devastation of infectious diseases, it is not surprising that efforts to treat them using a variety of substances began thousands of years ago when fragrant plants, herbs, and even molds were used for medicinal purposes. Early traders carried herbs, plants, and aromatic oils along the established routes of ancient civilizations, and many of these medicinal treatments are still used today. For instance, garlic (*Allium sativum*), which has been used for centuries to disinfect wounds and kill parasitic worms, was used by ancient Egyptians during the Nile Delta flood season when infestations of flies and mosquitoes were at their worst. For more than 2,500 years, traditional Chinese medicine has recommended ginger (*Zingiber officinale*) to soothe the digestive system and stop coughing. Licorice root (*Glycyrrhiza glabra*) was used thousands of years ago as a natural remedy for sore throats and coughs and is still the main ingredient in many cough formulations today. Primitive people in Central America used molds to treat infection, although the bacteria-killing mold penicillin would not be discovered for centuries. While these substances were known to relieve symptoms, the causes of disease were not understood until much later—not until well after the discovery of microscopic life.

The Discovery of "Animalcules"

Fifteenth-century physician Girolamo Frascatoro first voiced the notion that disease might be caused by invisible, "animate" particles. His ideas were not given serious attention, however, because the human eye could not see bacteria. Nearly two centuries later a Dutch cloth merchant named Antonie van Leeuwenhoek became fascinated looking through the magnifying lenses that he used to examine cloth. Inspired by the book *Micrographia*, an illustrated record of the microscopic observations of Oxford-educated scientist Robert Hooke, van Leeuwenhoek perfected the microscope and built more than 500 of them before he died at the remarkably old age of 90 in 1723. Using his microscopes, van Leeuwenhoek discovered even smaller organisms than the insects and cells that Hooke had observed. Van Leeuwenhoek called them "animalcules," and they included bacteria he had identified in dental plaque. Although van Leeuwenhoek is credited with officially discovering germs, the link between germs and disease would not be considered until more than a century later.

Germs and the Scientific Method

Although scientists had observed and documented the microscopic world, devastating infectious diseases continued to ravage the globe. For example, in the American colonies, the parasitic disease malaria was so common it was called "seasoning," referring to the fact that every newcomer had to survive it upon arriving. The impact of diseases like malaria, cholera, dysentery, and smallpox was so devastating that Cotton Mather, one of the early colonial leaders, noted in his diary that seeing dead children was "no more surprising than seeing a broken pitcher." In addition, diseases brought by the settlers decimated Native American populations, which had never been exposed to these unfamiliar germs.

Infectious disease played a key role in the development of the *scientific method*, a set of systematic rules and processes for experimentation. In 1721, Mather designed one of the world's earliest and most compelling scientific studies in an effort to test his theory that a process known as *variolation*—a precursor to vaccination—could prevent death by smallpox, a dreaded disease estimated to have killed one of every five people living in Boston in 1677 and disfiguring countless others. Using a thread, Mather collected pustules from people with nonfatal cases of smallpox and dried them, later placing the threads into cuts on a healthy recipient's skin. This typically resulted in a milder case of the disease, and Mather documented that natural infection killed 5 to 20 times more people than infection by variolation. Although the practice initially caused outrage in the scientific and medical community, Mather received the support of Benjamin Franklin, who lost his own son to smallpox and regretted his decision not to variolate.

Decades later, Englishman Edward Jenner noticed that British milkmaids who contracted cowpox—a much milder but similar disease—did not contract the deadly smallpox. In 1796, Jenner developed a vaccine derived from cowpox that was safer, led to general acceptance of vaccination, and ultimately resulted in the worldwide elimination of the disease. Jenner's first cowpox inoculation, which occurred a little more than 200 years ago, was one of the key precedents of the use of science in matters of health, and it helped to set the grand stage for research and development for one of our most significant weapons against germs today: vaccination.

The Age of Discovery

Up until the mid-1800s, however, scientists and doctors were still speculating about what caused disease. The prevailing theory was that disease occurred with no specific external cause, a theory called *spontaneous generation*. As the scientific method continued to develop, however, more evidence emerged about the existence of germs. This, in turn, resulted in a flurry of important scientific discoveries that led to the establishment of many of the foundations of modern medicine.

Improved Hospital Conditions

In 1847, Ignaz Semmelweis, an obstetrician in Vienna, asserted that doctors caused the spread of "childbed fever," a viral disease that caused the deaths of many women following childbirth. At that time, physicians did not wash their hands between deliveries and often would perform autopsies before attending to births. Semmelweis demonstrated that hand washing with a solution of chloride of lime before deliveries decreased the death rate from 18 percent to 2.5 percent. This discovery paved the way for the use of antiseptics in medicine and led Joseph Lister, a pioneering surgeon in a Scottish hospital, to develop the technique of applying carbolic acid solution to surgical instruments, wounds, and dressings. Lister's work revolutionized the processes of sterilization for surgery that continues today.

Improved Sanitation and Public Health

In 1848, a major outbreak of cholera killed more than 500 people within a few days in Golden Square, a section of the Soho district of London. While many theories about the cause of cholera existed, it took the perseverance of British physician John Snow to unravel the case of these deaths. By constructing a map showing the residences of those suffering from the disease, Snow realized that the deaths centered around a single water pump at Broad Street, a pump favored by many in the neighborhood for the taste and clarity of its water. Snow hypothesized that the water supply was the source of the problem.

When cholera struck again in 1854, Snow used the opportunity to test his theory. He tracked the cholera deaths, personally visiting the homes of each victim to ask about the source of its water. In the process, he learned that houses served by a single water system,

Southwark & Vauxhall Company (which filtered filthy sewage-contaminated water from the Thames River within London), had 8.5 times the number of cholera deaths as those served by the Lambeth Company's system (which also drew its water from the Thames, but about 10 miles upstream of London).

Snow single-handedly demonstrated that a microscopic agent that was too small to be caught in the filtering system used by the Southwark & Vauxhall Company caused cholera. His work not only led to dramatic changes in sanitation and water disinfection, but it laid the foundation for epidemiology, the scientific study of epidemics, that serves as a cornerstone of modern public health.

Improved Understanding of Germs and Medicine

French chemist Louis Pasteur, who had developed a heating process to kill the bacteria that caused wine to spoil, believed that if bacteria could cause spoilage, they could also cause disease. Pasteur and other scientists worked on experiments to test this theory. One of the most momentous of these took place in early May of 1881, when Pasteur visited a small farm just south of Paris. He inoculated several sheep, cows, and goats with a weakened form of the bacteria that causes anthrax, a devastating disease that frequently killed livestock. A separate group of animals was not inoculated. Several weeks later, Pasteur again visited the farm and vaccinated the first group with the weakened anthrax bacteria. On a third visit, Pasteur gave all of the animals a lethal injection of anthrax, both those that had been inoculated and those that had not.

A few days after the lethal injection, a crowd gathered to see the results of this groundbreaking experiment. As the onlookers watched, Pasteur led the vaccinated animals into a field, all of them in perfect health.

He then showed the group the animals that had not received vaccinations. Most of them were dead already, and the remainder died later that day. The experiment was a success. Not only had Pasteur proven that specific and isolated germs caused the disease but also he had found a way to prevent it by weakening those same germs and injecting them into a healthy animal.

Even though he isn't as famous as Pasteur is today, we must recognize the tremendous contributions of Robert Koch, a Nobel Prize–winning German physician and scientist who worked at the same time as Pasteur. Not only was Koch the first to link a specific organism to a specific disease through painstaking experimentation, but he established Koch's Postulates, a set of experimental steps that enabled countless other scientists to make this connection. Koch also invented new methods of growing bacteria on solid substances; in fact, one of his colleagues, Richard Petri, invented the familiar flat glass dish that so many of us have used in school science experiments.

These stunning discoveries contributed to the *germ theory of disease*, the scientific principle that disease does not occur spontaneously but is linked to specific organisms. This theory laid the groundwork not only for the medical treatment of disease, but also for an assortment of significant public health developments that have stood the test of time, including radical new measures to provide clean drinking water, milk, and food, to reduce the spread of infectious agents, and to safely dispose of waste products.

The Age of Miracles

This new understanding of germs led to many scientific discoveries, including the use of Gram's stain and other techniques to classify bacteria. These discoveries provided scientists with powerful tools to search for cures to the bacterial diseases that were still major killers throughout the world.

An Accidental Discovery

In the early 1900s, Scottish bacteriologist Alexander Fleming was one of very few doctors using salvarsan, an effective new arsenic-based drug developed by a German chemist to target *Treponema pallidum*, the bacterium causing the deadly disease syphilis. Fleming was later stationed in a battlefield hospital in World War I, where he was deeply distressed to see so many soldiers dying from infection. He searched for a drug that would treat surgical infections as safely and effectively as salvarsan had treated syphilis.

Back in his lab at St. Mary's Hospital in London, Fleming frequently conducted dozens of experiments at once. One day while he was cleaning up a variety of petri dishes that were stacked in a sink, he noticed something unusual. Mold was growing on many of the dishes, but in one of them all of the staph bacteria surrounding the mold had been killed. Fleming examined the mold and determined that it was *Penicillin notatum*. Although he published his findings, they generated little interest at the time.

Penicillin Rediscovered

In 1935, Howard Florey, an Australian pathologist working at Oxford University, came across Fleming's paper and organized a team of scientists to experiment with the penicillin mold. The team conducted further animal and human tests and found that penicillin cured a variety of bacterial infections. Although the drug was difficult and expensive to produce, England had entered World War II by this time, and the need for a drug to combat infection was critical. An agricultural research center in Illinois began to produce penicillin in large quantities, and others joined in once the United States entered the war. Some experts estimate that by the time the war ended, American companies were producing 650 billion units of penicillin each month.

The Age of Overkill

Only 4 years after drug companies began mass-producing penicillin in 1942, doctors began to see resistant strains of *Staphylococcus* in hospital settings. As the decades passed, more and more resistant strains emerged, and scientists raced to develop new antibiotics like methicillin to fight them. As reported in *Emerging Infectious Diseases*, worldwide, more than 95 percent of *S. aureus* infections today resist first-line antibiotics like penicillin or ampicillin, and more than 30 percent also resist second-line antibiotics like methicillin.

New Drugs' Frightening Failures

As strains of *S. aureus* became ever more resistant to first- and second-line antibiotics, an entirely new class of drugs called fluoroquinolones was introduced in 1980. Initially these drugs were highly successful, killing more than 95 percent of methicillin resistant strains. Yet within a single year, the CDC reported that 80 percent of those strains had become resistant to the fluoroquinolones.

A Note about Hospitals

Larger hospitals, those with more than 200 beds, are more likely to report antibiotic-resistant bacterial infections than smaller hospitals. Managed care facilities are less likely to have resistant strains of bacteria.

In fact, today more than 40 percent of staph infections are resistant to every drug except vancomycin. Given this drug's strength and its restricted status as a last resort for doctors to prescribe, it's terrifying to note that doctors and microbiologists are now beginning to report evidence of vancomycin-resistant *S. aureus* infections, as in a study published in the *New England Journal of Medicine*. In some cases, the vancomycin-resistant infections are proving to be untreatable, and patients are dying because of our inability to kill these infections.

Routine Resistance

While it's appalling to learn that drug-resistant bacteria kill vulnerable hospital patients, it's even more unnerving to realize that the resistant germs are limited neither to these locations nor to those who are already infirm. *Any of us can suddenly encounter a life-threatening bacterial illness at any time*, one that may not immediately respond to treatment. As I mentioned earlier, bacteria can adapt their genetic code to avoid destruction by antibiotics. The more often bacteria are exposed to an antibiotic, the greater the chance that the germs will figure out a way to outsmart that drug the next time they encounter it. Using such drugs, then, should logically be limited to the times when they are required, and they should be taken as directed.

Consequently, our over-reliance on antibiotics is of major global concern. In 1998, the Institute of Medicine estimated that the annual cost of treating antibiotic-resistant infections could be as high as $30 billion and that 20 to 50 percent of the more than 300 million annual prescriptions for antibiotics in the United States may not be medically justified. This overkill of medication often occurs because patients demand these drugs, usually for illnesses that are not bacterial at all. A study in

Antibiotics: A Modern Miracle

Antibiotics virtually eradicated infectious disease in the years following their introduction. According to the Centers for Disease Control and Prevention, the top three causes of death in the United States in 1900 were:

1. Pneumonia and influenza
2. Tuberculosis
3. Diarrhea, enteritis, and ulceration of the intestines

By 1996, these were replaced with:

1. Heart disease
2. Cancer
3. Stroke

By 1996, pneumonia and influenza had dropped to the sixth leading cause of death, and tuberculosis and diarrhea, enteritis, and ulceration of the intestines had dropped out of the top 10.

Archives of Family Medicine found that half of those who participated wanted an antibiotic prescription for care of cold symptoms that are often viral or nonbacterial in nature. Physicians may not explain that antibiotics will have no effect upon viral illnesses or explain the risks of antibiotic resistance to each and every patient. Some physicians may routinely prescribe antibiotics so they are not liable if the patient becomes ill with an infection at a later time.

It is amazing to think that once we receive antibiotics, many of us fail to take them as directed. We've all seen the label on our antibiotic prescription bottle: "Take all of this medication, even if your symptoms improve," or something to that effect. Yet many of us stop taking antibiotics once we feel better and stockpile the rest for later use, to save us a trip to the doctor. Failing to finish a course of antibiotics can leave a handful of bacteria behind—bacteria that have recently been exposed to the antibiotic and have learned to survive if they encounter it again.

The World Health Organization recently sounded the alarm that resistance to drugs is reaching a crisis point, with all major infections including tuberculosis, malaria, pneumonia, and diarrheal diseases slowly becoming resistant to existing drugs. Researchers have also expressed a growing concern that "routine" illnesses such as cystitis, bronchitis, and ear and sinus infections are becoming much more persistent and difficult to treat. Now a host of groundbreaking research is appearing, providing evidence that germs are winning the battle against antibiotics in many common ailments. Once again, overkill is to blame.

Take an unpleasant but non-life-threatening condition like acne, for example. For more than 20 years, antibiotics such as erythromycin and tetracycline have been used to treat moderate and severe forms of this annoying skin ailment. Resistance to these common antibiotics, however, has become an important threat to the use of these powerful drugs. In a study reported at the American Society for Microbiology's 2001 general meeting, researchers from the Karolinska Institute in Stockholm, Sweden, took bacterial skin samples from 99 patients with severe acne who had been receiving antibiotics for 2 to 6 months, and from 30 control subjects with severe acne who were receiving no antibiotics. They found that 28 percent of those receiving antibiotics harbored resistant strains of the acne-causing bacterium *Propionibacterium acnes*, as opposed to 6 percent of the control group, which means that those taking antibiotics were nearly five times more likely to harbor antibiotic-resistant organisms. These researchers recommended that doctors rethink the use of antibiotics in acne treatment and suggested using the drugs only as a last resort.

Similarly, scientists have found a possible explanation for why bladder infections caused by *E. coli* return in up to 30 percent of cases that appear to have been cured by antibiotics. A 2001 study suggests that bacteria may be able to survive antibiotic treatment by reverting to an inactive state. In the study, even after a full month of antibiotic treatment, an average of one-tenth of the original bacteria remained.

In a report published in *Archives of Internal Medicine* in 2001, scientists said they were perplexed by *Helicobacter pylori*, the ulcer-causing bacterium now believed to cause stomach cancer and that is typically treated with a complex, multidrug regimen including the drugs metronidazole and clarithromycin. The drugs had been successful in killing the bacteria in more than 80 percent of patients. New strains of *H. pylori*, however, appear to be becoming resistant to these drugs. In the study, researchers found that 35 percent of patients in the United States treated with the antibiotic metronidazole and 11 percent of those treated with clarithromycin harbored drug-resistant bacteria.

The list of common illnesses that are becoming resistant to our antibiotic arsenal is growing longer each year. Add to this our use and overuse of antibacterial products, which you'll read about below and in chapter 5, and it should be clear that we are on the brink of becoming deeply entrenched in the Age of Overkill.

Bacterial Resistance: A Crash Course

Throughout our discussion of the momentous advances in germ research and the precarious state in which we find ourselves today, I've used terms we've all heard or read about: antibiotics, bacterial resistance, and antibacterial products. But to truly understand how we got from the Age of Miracles to the Age of Overkill, here's a crash course in the compelling science that explains our current bacterial dilemma.

The Antibiotic Arsenal

Antibiotics were developed to target and kill bacteria without harming the cells in your body. They can be *bacteriocidal*, killing germs outright, or *bacteriostatic*, interfering with their ability to grow and reproduce. Antibiotics do this in several ways: by preventing bacteria from producing adequate cell walls for their protection, by interfering with bacteria's ability to synthesize or metabolize substances they need for survival, or by blocking bacteria's ability to reproduce. The first antibiotics, like penicillin, were *narrow-spectrum*, killing bacteria only of certain types, but later developments included antibiotics like vancomycin, *broad-spectrum* agents that kill a wider variety of bacteria and allow doctors to treat patients with infections caused by unknown bacteria.

How Bacteria Fight Back

Germs are survivors—after all, they've been on the planet longer than any other form of life. They've learned how to adapt to a variety of threats, including antibiotics. Here are some of the ways that bacteria outsmart their once-effective antibacterial foes:

- Some bacteria produce enzymes that neutralize the drug.
- If they sense a medication that is harmful to them, some bacteria can change the permeability of their cell walls to prevent the drug from entering.
- Bacteria can create substances that in effect escort the antibiotic out of the cell if it happens to get in unnoticed.
- Some antibiotics target a particular part of the bacteria; in order

to survive, the bacteria simply change that part of their anatomy so that the drug no longer recognizes it.

Bacteria are continually reacting and evolving, and it's not uncommon for them to become multidrug-resistant, which means they can outsmart more than one type of antibiotic.

The Bacterial Learning Curve

Bacteria can evolve rapidly, so it's possible for a single bacterium to make the changes described above and itself become resistant to drugs. But some bacteria acquire resistance by learning trade secrets about how to beat antibiotics from other bacteria. This occurs by a variety of means: through plasmids, free-floating pieces of DNA that can contain instructions for resistance to several antibiotics; through the remains of dead bacteria; or during transformation, where two bacteria can transfer pieces of DNA to each other.

Bacterial Resistance and Our Food Supply

Bacterial resistance can also occur when antibiotics are added in low doses to the food of cows, pigs, and poultry, a common practice in the United States today. By some estimates, nearly half of the antibiotics used in our country might be used for livestock, not only to combat disease but also to promote growth. Though the consensus is that human antibiotic abuse is the chief contributor to the resistance problem, top experts in this field recognize a potential link between drug-resistant bacteria and antibiotic use in livestock food. Finland, Sweden, and Denmark have eliminated the practice of feeding drugs to animals to promote growth, but the practice continues elsewhere, including here.

Add to these concerns the dangers posed by the "normal" bacteria in our food. With increased globalization and population growth, our demand for fresh produce and other imported foods opens the door to an increasing array of germs from other countries. Changes in food production practices may also increase the amount and types of these germs.

Antibacterials: A False Sense of Security

Manufacturers continue to meet consumer demands and capitalize on consumer germophobia by flooding the market with a dizzying array of antibacterial products. While some scientists warn that these products are contributing to the global resistance crisis, consumers are hesitant to give them up.

Triclosan, one of the most common antibacterial ingredients, has been used in soap since the 1960s. Today it's starting to be used in everything from food-storage containers to high chairs. In fact, you might have to look carefully to find soap without antibacterial agents, since so many of the soap products on the market now contain germ killers. The reason for this is simple supply and demand: Americans now spend more than $400 million a year just on antibacterial hand soaps! If this sounds like overkill, you're beginning to get the idea.

Researchers originally believed that triclosan worked like alcohol, bleach, and other antiseptic cleaners by simply breaking down the cell walls of bacteria. Now they've hypothesized that triclosan may act more like a broad-spectrum antibiotic, targeting and destroying an enzyme that bacteria need for survival. Scientists are beginning to examine triclosan in the laboratory to see if it creates significant resistance. In an experiment at Colorado State University in Fort Collins, as reported in *Antimicrobial Agents and Chemotherapy* in 2001, exposure to triclosan caused bacteria to become resistant to several common antibiotics. In addition, studies indicate that triclosan may not be effective at killing certain bacteria, including *Streptococcus pneumoniae*, the bacteria that cause pneumonia and some cases of meningitis.

Although antibacterial products containing triclosan are believed to be topically harmless to humans, this chemical can be stored in body fat and can cause damage to organs if it reaches toxic levels within the body. Many medical experts suggest that the extensive use of antibacterial products is overkill and that these products should be reserved for those individuals at high risk or for cleaning jobs that particularly warrant their use.

Antibacterials and Our Children

Antibacterial products raise another concern: Some scientists now theorize that raising children in squeaky-clean environments can compromise their immune systems, resulting in imbalances in immune response. This theory, called the Hygiene Hypothesis, is one of many being proposed to explain the observed increases in allergy and asthma. Statistics from the National Heart, Lung and Blood Institute show that asthma rates in children under 4 years of age have more than doubled since 1980. Research is ongoing, but preliminary findings in some studies suggest that there are fewer instances of asthma and allergies in children who grew up on farms, began daycare at an early age, or received fewer antibiotics at an early age.

Scientists are examining these and a variety of other factors that may impact children's developing immune systems, including a decline in breastfeeding, an increase in indoor play, and the effect of exposure to pets and secondhand smoke. They warn that the full effect of germ overkill on our children may not become evident for another 10 years or more. I'll talk more about the Hygiene Hypothesis in chapter 4, and we'll explore the ways you can safeguard and optimize your children's health.

Ushering in a New Age: The Age of Risk Management

Now that you understand how the Age of Overkill developed, I'm certain you'll agree that the responsibility for resolving this crisis falls to each of us. We need to move beyond the false belief that killing all germs is desirable or even possible. We need to reduce our dependence on antibiotics and antibacterial products and use them only when they're appropriate. We need to understand that medical science can't resolve this problem without our help; each of us must take personal charge of our own health.

For the past decade, I've been studying health-risk issues in depth. During that time I've been distressed to see the medical and public health establishments scramble to solve this problem and at the same time to get information out to the public. That's why I wanted to write this book—to provide you with accurate, cutting-edge information such as how a few simple steps taken early in an illness can protect your health; what to do when a family member becomes ill; and how to demand the proper treatments when you need them because when used properly, antibiotics can save your life.

Above all, it's important for you to feel confident that you are doing all you can to stay infection-free and to live an active, healthy life. So, if you are ready to begin, sharpen a pencil and turn to chapter 2, where you'll find the questionnaire that will help us all to enter a new age—the Age of Risk Management.

2

CALCULATING YOUR RISK QUOTIENT

As an assistant professor of risk analysis and decision science at Harvard University School of Public Health, my job is to identify, analyze, and assess health risks—all types of health risks. When I give speeches about managing risk, I usually begin by sharing a partial list of the hazards I've faced up to that point in the day. This might include the possibility of falling in the shower, being electrocuted by my blow dryer, choking on my breakfast, or getting into a car accident. I could expand this list indefinitely—you'll notice that I haven't even mentioned germs yet!

Before you accuse me of being paranoid, let me explain that as a risk analyst I focus on probability—the chance that something really will happen, and I also consider the consequences. How serious is the risk? What's at stake? Are you risking death or severe illness, or just a day of bed rest? Whatever health hazard you can imagine, I can examine it, crunch some numbers on it, and explore ways to reduce the risk.

Perhaps the easiest way for me to explain risk analysis is to compare it to detective work. In mystery novels, the detective possesses a basic understanding of the situation at hand, but he also asks myriad questions to learn the solid facts about the case. While a detective looks for evidence linking a suspect to a crime, a risk analyst looks for evidence linking a factor—an element of our lives that impacts us—to a health outcome—a real positive or negative influence on our health. For example, risk analysts might try to learn whether a factor like frequent hand washing is associated with a health outcome such as a decreased risk of food poisoning, or whether antibacterial products are associated with reduced illnesses in young children, or whether crowded dormitory conditions are associated with increased episodes of strep throat or bronchitis.

Just as detectives rely on their understanding of human behavior to assemble a case, risk analysts must also understand people and their behaviors. In my work, I examine the situations, lifestyles, and behaviors that place people at a variety of risks, such as eating undercooked meat, having unprotected sex, or stockpiling medicine to avoid a trip to the doctor. Then I assess the chances that people will experience injury, disease, or even death as a result of these behaviors.

You might think that a bacteriologist would be the best person to advise you about your bacterial risks, but that isn't the case. While their work is vital in the fight against germs that threaten us, most bacteriologists focus intently on one aspect of germ life: a particular bacterium, the way it performs a certain function, or how a specific action varies

Risky Business

Each of the following lifestyle habits might negatively affect your immune function and make you more susceptible to illness when exposed to bacterial infection. Work to change these, try to avoid them, or make allowances for their impact on your health.

- Too little sleep
- Negative attitude
- Repressed feelings
- Sense of worthlessness
- Poor diet
- Few fresh fruits and vegetables
- Extreme exercise
- Sedentary lifestyle
- No social support
- Recent job loss or lack of employment
- Job dissatisfaction
- Shift work
- Recent death of a loved one
- Caregiving to a chronically ill person
- Marital separation and/or divorce
- Exposure to environmental pollutants
- Overexposure to sunlight
- Cigarette smoking
- Heavy alcohol use
- Long-term medication usage

among different bacterial types. Most bacteriologists are not trained to assess public health risks, and it's generally not part of their job descriptions to look up from their microscopes and tell the rest of us how to deal with every type of germ in our environments.

That's where my specialty comes in. Like many scientists, I start by reviewing the most up-to-date, reliable research literature available. I've read up on every aspect of bacteria—the benign and beneficial as well as those that can harm us. I've studied the published opinions of a variety of experts, including bacteriologists, epidemiologists, toxicologists, physicians, and psychologists, in order to learn all I can about how we transmit germs, how we control and beat them, and how they're learning to fight back. I've assembled all of these pieces to form the most complete picture of the problem possible, linking the factors to the outcomes and allowing us to identify ways to reduce our risks of bacterial illnesses.

As I've mentioned before, no single approach will solve the problem. What is called for is an individualized approach that considers all of the bacterial risks in your life. To help you determine the best course of action for you and your family, I've done the next best thing to consulting with you in person. I've designed the Personal Health Risk Profile, a 50-item questionnaire that analyzes your risk factors for infection. You'll see that some of these factors are unavoidable aspects of life, such as your family characteristics, while others are factors you can control, leading to improved health. Once you've completed the questionnaire, you'll calculate your Risk Quotient, a number between 1 and 5 that you'll use throughout the rest of the book.

But before I take you through the process of calculating your Risk Quotient, it's important for you to understand that there is no such thing as zero risk. We all have some probability—no matter how miniscule—of becoming ill and possibly even dying from exposure to bacteria. And it is not simply your exposure to germs that determines whether you will get sick; the daily choices you make play a key role in determining your risk level. Other things matter too, including your overall health, your diet, your lifestyle habits and stress level, and even your psychological state. (Revealing studies in the emerging field of psychoneuroimmunology now focus on the mind and body being interconnected, and in many cases your emotional state can determine your physical well-being.)

Your Personal Health Risk Profile

The Personal Health Risk Profile contains 50 questions—10 questions in each of five categories:

1. Personal and family characteristics
2. Current health status
3. Personal hygiene and home care practices
4. Food preferences and preparation
5. Occupation and leisure activities

For those of you who experience test anxiety, please realize that *this is not a test*. There are no right or wrong answers. The questions simply provide an eye-opening opportunity for you to assess your own risk of illness, as well as to identify those areas you can work on to improve your overall health. Following the questions, you'll find instructions on tallying your score to determine your numerical Risk Quotient, or RQ. Your RQ will range from 1 (a *low* level of risk) to 5 (a *high* level of risk). I will refer to your RQ throughout the remaining chapters of the book in order to individualize recommendations regarding medical care, child care, home hygiene, food preparation, and special situations such as living with a chronic illness or living in a dormitory or long-term care facility. My goal is to help you make your own better germ-related health choices, while respecting your preferences, not to make those choices for you.

The best way to approach the Personal Health Risk Profile is to get a piece of paper, number it from 1 to 50, and record your answers (*a* through *e*) so that at the end you can easily compute your Risk Quotient using the key. After you've scored your RQ, give the test to your spouse and kids and tally their scores. By doing this, you will get a clear picture of your own risk as well as your family's. Then, by following the strategies that I share in chapters 3 through 7, you can develop a personalized program to avoid illness from exposure to bacteria and learn to intelligently treat the illnesses you do get, without immediately resorting to antibiotics if you don't need them. Ultimately, this should help you improve your quality of life.

Personal and Family Characteristics

1. How many people currently reside in your home?
   (a) 1
   (b) 2
   (c) 3
   (d) 4
   (e) 5 or more

If you live in a shared apartment, then count the number of people in your unit (or the number of people who share your kitchen). If you live in a dormitory or other institutional setting, select (e), even if you have your own room.

2. How many pets share your household?
   (a) None
   (b) Outdoor pets
   (c) One indoor pet
   (d) One indoor/outdoor pet
   (e) Multiple indoor/outdoor pets

Note that an outdoor pet is one that never comes inside, such as a farm dog, and an indoor pet is one that never goes outside. Most people have indoor/outdoor pets, even if the animal spends most of its time either inside or outside. Generally, the more time the pet spends in your house, the greater its potential impact on your health.

3. How old is your home?

(a) Less than 5 years

(b) 5 to 10 years

(c) 10 or more years

(d) 20 or more years

(e) 50 or more years

4. How many years have you lived in your current home?

(a) Less than 5

(b) 5 to 10

(c) 10 or more

(d) 20 or more

(e) 50 or more

5. How many people live in your city?

(a) Fewer than 1,000

(b) More than 1,000

(c) More than 10,000

(d) More than 100,000

(e) More than 1 million

6. What is the source of water for your home for all water uses including drinking?

(a) Bottled water for drinking (select this answer even if you use other water sources for other uses)

(b) Ground water from private well source

(c) Ground water from city source

(d) Surface water from city source (select this answer if your city uses both ground and surface water)

(e) Collected rainwater or a private surface water source (select [d] if you are certain this water is disinfected and/or filtered to remove harmful pathogens)

If you don't know the answer to this question, call your city water department or local department of health. Ask about the water quality in your area and where you should turn for information about water advisories. In general, surface water is more likely to become contaminated with harmful bacteria than ground water, but most water in the United States is treated and chlorinated to kill bacteria.

7. How well do you maintain your heating, ventilation, and air conditioning systems?
   (a) Excellent maintenance (change all filters and clean all heating and air conditioning systems as recommended)
   (b) Good maintenance (periodically change filters and clean systems, but not quite as often as recommended)
   (c) No heating or cooling systems used so no maintenance performed; open windows for ventilation
   (d) Poor maintenance (rarely change filters and clean systems)
   (e) Never concerned with air quality and perform no maintenance on any systems
8. How do you tend to greet friends when you see them?
   (a) With a smile, but no touching
   (b) Handshake
   (c) Hug only
   (d) Kiss only
   (e) Hug and kiss
9. Within the past year, how many "safe" sexual partners have you had?
   (a) 0
   (b) 1
   (c) 2
   (d) 3 or 4
   (e) 5 or more

If you have had unprotected sexual intercourse with anyone in the past year, select (e), unless you are in a committed monogamous relationship and you are certain that your partner has also been sexually active only with you, in which case select (b). For our purposes, count incidences of oral sex.

10. How many people living with you spend part of their day around young children?

(a) 0

(b) 1, me

(c) 2 or more, including me

(d) 1 of my children

(e) 2 or more of my children

If you have young children living with you, then answer (b) or (c). If your young children are also around other kids—for example, in day care, play groups, preschool, or elementary school—choose either (d) or (e).

Current Health Status

11. How long has it been since you last saw a doctor for a routine physical exam?

(a) 1 year or less

(b) 2 years

(c) 3 years

(d) 4 years

(e) 5 or more years

12. How many times have you been ill enough to stay home for at least 1 day in the past 12 months?

(a) 0

(b) 1

(c) 2

(d) 3

(e) More than 3

13. How many times have you taken antibiotics during the past 12 months?

(a) 0

(b) 1

(c) 2

(d) 3

(e) More than 3

14. When you take antibiotics, do you follow the doctor's orders by taking the medication at the right time as directed and by finishing the entire prescription?

(a) Always

(b) Usually

(c) Sometimes

(d) Rarely

(e) Never

15. What is your current immunization status?

(a) Fully immunized

(b) Almost fully immunized

(c) Partially immunized

(d) Very limited immunizations

(e) Never immunized

Select (c) if you are unsure of your immunization status or if you haven't kept your immunizations up-to-date—if, for example, you have not had a tetanus booster in the past 10 years.

16. What, if any, medical conditions do you have that make you particularly likely to become ill?

(a) None

(b) Nothing myself, but I live with someone whose immune system is compromised or has a chronic disease or another condition and who is often ill

(c) Condition other than chronic disease or compromised immune system

(d) Chronic disease

(e) Compromised immune system

Several factors can weaken, or compromise, your immune system, including an inherited condition, treatments such as chemotherapy, immune diseases such as HIV or AIDS, and other illnesses like cirrhosis or severe diabetes.

If you are unsure about how to answer this question, check with your physician.

17. Have you been hospitalized or in institutional care?

(a) Never

(b) Rarely or only for delivery of a baby or elective surgery

(c) Occasionally, but not recently (choose this option if you have experienced regular hospitalizations in the past but not within the last few years)

(d) Regularly, including recently

(e) Recently or currently

18. How much do you smoke?

(a) Never

(b) Former smoker (permanently quit)

(c) Occasionally

(d) Regularly

(e) Heavily

19. How frequently do you drink alcohol?

(a) Never

(b) Occasionally

(c) Regularly, but in moderate amounts (one drink a day)

(d) Regularly, not in moderate amounts (two to three drinks a day)

(e) Heavily (more than three drinks a day)

Count each can of beer, glass of wine, or shot of hard liquor as a single drink.

20. How do you rate your current overall health?

(a) Excellent

(b) Very good

(c) Good

(d) Fair

(e) Poor

Personal Hygiene and Home Care Practices

21. How often do you wash your hands after using the bathroom or changing a child's diaper?

(a) Always

(b) Usually

(c) Sometimes

(d) Rarely

(e) Never

22. How often do you bathe or shower?

(a) More than once a day

(b) Daily

(c) 2 or 3 times a week

(d) Weekly

(e) Rarely

23. How often is your house thoroughly cleaned, including dusted and vacuumed?

(a) 2 or more times a week

(b) Weekly

(c) Monthly

(d) Annually

(e) Never

24. How often do you use antibacterial products for cleaning?

(a) When needed (choose this option if you use these products only in the "hot spots" of your home, where you know they are necessary)

(b) Sometimes

(c) Usually

(d) Always

(e) Never

25. How often do you keep raw or undercooked meats, poultry, or fish completely isolated from other foods and cooking items (including surfaces, cutting boards, serving dishes, and utensils) in your kitchen?

(a) Always

(b) Usually

(c) Sometimes

(d) Rarely

(e) Never

26. How meticulous are you about disinfecting the cooking items mentioned in question 25 that may have become contaminated in your kitchen?

(a) Very meticulous (disinfect immediately)

(b) Somewhat meticulous (disinfect as part of regular cleaning, 2 or more times a week)

(c) Not particularly meticulous (disinfect as part of weekly kitchen cleaning)

(d) Not at all meticulous (disinfect infrequently)

(e) Never disinfect these items

27. How often do you observe pests (including rats, mice, cockroaches, ants, or other creatures) in you home?

(a) Never

(b) Occasionally

(c) Monthly

(d) Weekly

(e) Daily

28. How often do you exterminate pests in your home?

(a) When needed to deal with a problem (choose this option if extermination is not needed)

(b) Monthly

(c) Annually

(d) Once every few years

(e) Never

29. How well is moisture controlled in your home?

(a) Never had a moisture problem

(b) Occasional leaks, but no permanent water damage

(c) Single incident of water damage within the last year that has been repaired

(d) Recurring incidents of water damage that have regularly been repaired (for example, basement flooding)

(e) Obvious constant moisture problem and visibly stained areas that have not been repaired

30. How do you rate your overall personal hygiene and home care practices?

(a) Excellent

(b) Very good

(c) Good

(d) Fair

(e) Poor

Food Preferences and Preparation

31. How often do you inspect meats, poultry, or fish for obvious signs of contamination and seek information about their freshness when you buy them (for example, by asking the butcher and by checking the dates on the package)?

(a) Always

(b) Usually

(c) Sometimes

(d) Rarely

(e) Never

If you are a vegetarian, this question applies to your main source of protein (e.g., tofu).

32. How often do you handle raw or undercooked meats, poultry, or fish?

(a) Never

(b) Occasionally

(c) Monthly

(d) Weekly

(e) Daily

33. How often do you eat raw or rare (undercooked) meats, poultry, or fish?

(a) Never

(b) Occasionally

(c) Monthly

(d) Weekly

(e) Daily

34. How often do you wash fruits and vegetables before eating them?

(a) Always

(b) Usually

(c) Sometimes

(d) Rarely

(e) Never

35. How would you describe your overall diet with respect to the variety of foods you eat?

(a) Highly varied

(b) Somewhat varied

(c) Somewhere in the middle (not varied or limited)

(d) Somewhat limited

(e) Very limited

36. Do you like hot (spicy) food, or foods containing onions, garlic, or lemon?

(a) Yes, always

(b) Yes, usually

(c) Yes, sometimes

(d) Yes, but rarely

(e) No, never

37. How often do you eat food prepared away from your home?

(a) Never

(b) Monthly

(c) Weekly

(d) 2 or 3 times a week

(e) Daily

38. How often do you eat imported foods or in authentic ethnic restaurants?

(a) Never

(b) Occasionally

(c) Monthly

(d) Weekly

(e) Daily

39. How quickly do you eat leftover foods?

(a) Never eat them

(b) Within 1 day

(c) Within 2 days

(d) Within 3 days

(e) Whenever I get to them

40. How do you rate your overall food safety practices?

(a) Excellent

(b) Very good

(c) Good

(d) Fair

(e) Poor

In answering this question, consider how well you know the USDA and FDA recommendations for food safety. Also think about your training in food safety by the people who taught you to cook. Was food safety emphasized?

Occupation and Leisure Activities

41. How often do your social or leisure activities put you in contact with people who are frequently ill?

(a) Never

(b) Occasionally

(c) Monthly

(d) Weekly

(e) Daily

42. How often do you travel out of the country?

(a) Never

(b) Rarely

(c) Occasionally

(d) Frequently, but always to the same place

(e) Frequently, all over the world

43. How often do you stay away from your home (for example, in hotels or with friends)?

(a) Never

(b) Rarely

(c) Occasionally

(d) Frequently

(e) Away from home more than half the year

44. How often are any of the people with whom you closely work ill?

(a) Never

(b) Occasionally

(c) Monthly

(d) Weekly

(e) Daily

45. How much stress do you feel on your job or at home?

(a) None

(b) A little

(c) Occasional

(d) Often

(e) Constant

46. How many hours do you spend on vigorous exercise (half-hour periods of strength training or aerobic exercise such as walking or bicycling) in a typical week?

(a) More than 15

(b) 10 to 15

(c) 5 to 10

(d) 1 to 5

(e) Less than 1

47. On average, how often do you work in a garden or on a farm over the course of the year?

(a) Never

(b) Occasionally

(c) Monthly

(d) Weekly

(e) Daily

48. How many hours of leisure do you average per week?

(a) More than 15

(b) 10 to 15

(c) 5 to 10

(d) 1 to 5

(e) Less than 1

Leisure for our purposes means time to enjoy yourself and relax, including only the time spent with family and friends that is truly relaxing and any times that you make a conscious effort to relax (even if this is while you drive your car).

49. How satisfied are you with the work you do?

(a) Generally very satisfied

(b) Generally somewhat satisfied

(c) Sometimes (b), sometimes (d), depending on the day

(d) Generally somewhat dissatisfied

(e) Generally very dissatisfied

50. How much control do you feel you have about the risks you take in your life and about your own ability to control your health?

(a) A lot of control

(b) Some control

(c) Little control

(d) Very little control

(e) No control

Figuring Your Risk Quotient

Now that you've answered the questions, it's time to interpret your score so you can see where you fit on the risk spectrum. Your Risk Quotient will help you figure out your optimal risk management strategies so that you can avoid overkill—going too far—while encouraging you to make sure that you are doing enough to combat harmful bacteria. Bear in mind that I'd have to meet with you individually to get *all* of the complex information needed to give you a complete picture of your risk. Here we're aiming for a relatively simple means of tallying a score that will be easy to understand and apply.

Use the following key to assign a numerical value to each of your letter responses:

(a) = 1	(d) = 4
(b) = 2	(e) = 5
(c) = 3	

Now add up all of the numbers to compute your total score. Next, divide your total score by 50 and round this answer to the nearest whole number (for instance, a 2.4 is a 2, a 3.7 is a 4). If your score is greater than 5, round it down to 5. The whole number that you end up with represents your Risk Quotient (RQ).

What Your RQ Means

Risk Quotient 1: Congratulations! You are in excellent health and have safe and healthy lifestyle habits. The bacteria in your environment pose relatively little risk to your health. You have the luxury of taking a more laid back approach to these risks than most people. Still, remember that there is no such thing as zero risk, and you still play a critical role in avoiding overkill. Continue to read to see what you might do to maintain optimal health and well-being and to take actions to prevent and relieve bacterial illness.

Risk Quotient 2: Although you are on the right track with your health and lifestyle habits and have a relatively small risk of bacterial illness, there are still some health, lifestyle, and hygiene areas that you might want to evaluate. Read on to find innovative ways to maintain optimal health and manage the bacteria in your daily life.

Risk Quotient 3: Because you have a moderate risk of bacterial illness, the information in chapters 3 through 7 will guide you toward healthier living and offer sound, self-care remedies for treating an assortment of bacterial ailments. I will help you to understand why it's important to be proactive and change negative lifestyle habits with prevention measures so that your chance of becoming ill is greatly reduced.

Risk Quotient 4: You have a relatively high risk of bacterial illness. Even though you may not feel at risk, consider implementing some of the strategies and self-care techniques I recommend in chapters 3 through 7 to reduce your chance of getting bacterial illnesses and to effectively treat them when they do occur.

Risk Quotient 5: You are at the highest risk for getting bacterial illness. Work with your doctor to address any health problems you can control. Then read chapters 3 through 6 to see the specific strategies I suggest to avoid illness. Also review chapter 7, which gives special instructions for high-risk individuals to further decrease their chances of bacterial infection.

Beyond Your RQ

Now that you know your own RQ for bacterial infection, you're ready to discover what you can do to help protect yourself from illness. But before we proceed, I want to make a few pertinent points about the Personal Health Risk Profile and your Risk Quotient.

First, even though each question received equal weight in computing your RQ, some of the questions are much more important in predicting your risk for bacterial infection than others. For example, question 9 (the one that asks about sex) is critical, as sexually transmitted diseases continue to steal years of life from both men and women and rob them of the chance to have children. I would be remiss as a public health expert if I didn't emphasize that the HIV virus that causes AIDS should be the ultimate fear for those who are practicing unsafe sex. AIDS is now considered to be a disease of our youth in America. The public health community is losing in its prevention efforts that must compete with sexual images and messages that pervade American popular culture—a culture that virtually ignores the risks of sexual activity and encourages sex among young people. If you've seen the movie *American Pie* or talked candidly with many high school students, you're likely to learn the surprising fact that for them, "third base" probably means oral sex. A study in the *Journal of the American Medical Association* in 1999 showed that Americans have widely divergent views on what constitutes sex. The reason public health officials have been alerted about this trend is that doctors in California are reporting seeing teenage girls who have gonorrhea infections in their throats that must be treated with antibiotics, and gonorrhea is becoming resistant to the antibiotics used to treat it. I'm not belittling or ignoring the benefits of sex, but it's important to appreciate the risks, too, and to realize that now the risks extend beyond pregnancy and AIDS. The risks include syphilis, gonorrhea, human papillomaviruses (HPV) that can cause cervical cancer, and other sexually transmitted diseases, many of which continue to become more difficult to treat. In contrast, question 5 (the one that asks how many people live in your town) is less important. The relationship between urban areas, rural areas, and bacterial risks is still unclear, although we do know that the more people who live near you the more likely you'll be in proximity to someone who is spreading "bad" germs.

Second, your RQ is not a definitive measure of your risk. It is intended to give you a rough sense of where you are on the spectrum so you have a guide for individualizing how you should manage your risks. If you find that you have one score and another member of your family has a different score, then for family and home issues assume the higher of the two scores. For instance, if your RQ is 2 and your spouse's is 4, take the higher score of 4 for your household and follow through with the recommended strategies for that RQ.

Third, no matter what Risk Quotient you have, you can use this book as a resource to make the changes necessary to lower your risk and avoid the problem of antibiotic resistance in your own home. For example, if your RQ is high because your food hygiene is not up to par, use the suggestions in chapters 5 and 6 to improve in this area. Keep in mind that your lifestyle choices and habits matter a great deal in determining your Risk Quotient and the outcome—your health status. If your choices, preferences, or situation change significantly, then reassess your Risk Quotient.

When you review the questionnaire again, ask yourself why a certain answer to a question might increase your score. For example, in question 1 I ask for the number of people you live with. As you might guess, as the number of people you live with increases, your risks of exposure to viral and bacterial diseases increase. Clearly, this is an example of something that you probably can't change, depending on your situation. (And I have no interest in breaking up families in the name of lower bacterial risks!) Another example would be in question 2, where I ask you about your pets. Household pets are associated with increased risks of asthma, and they are also effective at spreading germs, particularly in their feces. The type or types of pets you have also matter with respect to how you manage the risks, even though that is not reflected in the question. For example, the issues associated with preventing transmission of disease are different for a bird than for a dog; cats may be a serious health concern if you're pregnant. Talk to your veterinarian about diseases that you can get from your pets, and always wash your hands thoroughly before and after touching them.

Fourth, your bacterial risk is only one kind of risk in your life. As a health-risk analyst, I can tell you of innumerable risks that you could manage and how you should be aware of the concept of benefits. Benefits are rewards you get that have a positive, personal value and that might make taking risks worthwhile. I know that swimming in a lake or pool could mean that I'll be exposed to some bacteria in the water. But as a person who loves to swim, the benefits of being in a pool exercising and having fun may far outweigh any risks.

Another concept you must understand is that of risk trade-offs you might incur by taking a particular action. They can involve other bacterial risks or other types of risks altogether, and they are a part of risk management. You should also recognize that you have a limited number of practical strategies for managing germs and tools available to kill germs and that there are benefits and risks for all of these. One goal of this book is to help you appreciate, understand, and think about the trade-offs so that you may strike the healthy balance that's right for you and your family, considering your own values and preferences.

Finally, some special situations warrant additional considerations, no matter what your Risk Quotient, and these are covered in-depth in chapter 7. For example, some reports associate the increase in preschoolers' doctor's visits for ear infections over the past decade to the increased use of daycare facilities. We must address how the poorly developed hygiene habits of young children combined with the close quarters of the center allow disease-causing microbes to flourish and spread so quickly. College students who live in dormitories or other shared accommodations and military personnel who reside in crowded barracks represent other special populations at risk for infectious diseases. People on chemotherapy, transplant recipients taking drugs to suppress their immune function, and other immune compromised individuals are at greater risk of infection than the normal population. Nurseries in hospitals and long-term care facilities for the elderly are other reservoirs of harmful bacteria, as evidenced by their elevated rates of infection and death.

Germ-Tackling Tools

A variety of tools exist to reduce the health risks in our environment. Although medical science has uncovered many ways to prevent bacterial illness, these methods fall into 10 basic categories:

1. Hand washing: The CDC and other public health experts agree that hand washing is the single most important means of preventing the spread of infection, yet a study conducted in 2000 by the American Society for Microbiology revealed that about one-third of Americans using public restrooms in five major cities didn't wash their hands before leaving. Our hands come into daily contact with a multitude of contaminated surfaces, and when we touch our faces, germs can enter our bodies through our eyes, nose, and mouth. We can also transmit those germs to others by shaking hands or handling items that are then touched by others. Proper hand washing is sufficient to remove most bacteria, and here's how to do it:

- Run the water until it's warm; wet your hands thoroughly.
- Apply enough plain soap to work up a good lather.
- Rub your hands together for 15 to 20 seconds, washing both sides of each hand, the spaces between each finger, and around rings, paying special attention to the areas around fingernails. (Whenever you have the time, it's a good idea to use a nailbrush, as bacteria tend to hide under your nails, and keep your nails trimmed.)
- Rinse your hands thoroughly.
- Turn off the faucet without touching it if you can because bacteria thrive on faucet handles. (Depending on the type of faucet, you can use a paper towel or maybe your elbow.)
- Dry your hands thoroughly with a clean cloth towel, a paper towel, or an air dryer.
- If possible, don't use your hands to open the bathroom door (either push it open with your shoulder or use a paper towel to turn the knob).

Wash your hands frequently throughout the day—before and after you eat, after using the bathroom, after gardening, before and after sex, and after handling any potential contaminants like raw meat, unwashed vegetables, dirty diapers, or garbage.

2. Antiseptics: Antiseptics are substances that destroy disease-causing microorganisms, typically by breaking down cell walls. These include well-known antiseptics like alcohol, hydrogen peroxide, and chlorine bleach.

3. Avoidance: One of the simplest ways to avoid infection is to avoid the bacteria that cause it. For example, you might avoid kissing a grandchild with a bad cold, or you might avoid touching your face—a very common way of picking up colds and flu. (This includes avoiding putting your fingers in your mouth and not biting your nails.)

4. Barriers: Placing a barrier between yourself and the world is a very effective way to avoid germs. You may have noticed that paper toilet seat covers are becoming more common in public restrooms. Use them! Other effective barriers include wearing sandals in locker rooms and saunas to avoid direct contact with the floor and condoms during sexual activity to prevent the exchange of bacteria and viruses.

5. Preventing moisture: Bacteria thrive in moist environments, so preventing moisture is a great way to keep germs at bay. If you use a bar soap, make sure to keep it on a rack so it drains and doesn't sit in a pool of water. Kitchen sponges and towels should also be kept on racks when they aren't used to allow them to dry as quickly as possible.

6. Boiling: The process of boiling kills many harmful bacteria. People at high risk of infection can boil pots of water and use them for drinking. When sponges are placed in the microwave, the water they contain is effectively boiled off and most of the bacteria they harbor are neutralized. And while the water in your tap doesn't quite reach the boiling point—and it shouldn't, for very practical safety reasons—laundering clothes in hot water and then drying them thoroughly kills many bacteria and is a good way to keep kitchen towels, bed linens, and bath towels as clean as possible.

7. Temperature control: The bacteria in our environments tend to thrive in temperatures between 40° and 140° F. Refrigeration prevents many bacteria from growing, but most of us don't know exactly how cold our refrigerators are. It's a good idea to keep a thermometer inside the fridge and make sure it reads below 40°. In addition, heating food to the appropriate temperatures kills many of the bacteria and other microbes that cause food-borne illness. A good meat thermometer is a must and should be used in the thickest part of the meat to determine whether the interior temperature is high enough.

8. Ventilation: Modern heating and air conditioning systems are designed for energy efficiency, but they recirculate germ-filled air. In confined spaces like airplanes and small offices, you're exposed to a higher concentration of disease-causing microbes. It's important to change the filters in your heaters and air conditioners often and to ventilate your home using fresh air as often as possible.

9. Vaccination: Injection with inactive germs encourages our immune system to respond without causing us severe illness. The immune system "remembers" that type of germ and will attack and kill it very quickly if it encounters it again in the future.

10. Antibiotics and antibacterials: While antiseptics like alcohol and bleach simply break up bacterial cell walls, antibiotics and antibacterials generally prevent bacteria from building their cell walls properly, interfere with their ability to make or metabolize substances for their survival, or prevent them from reproducing. While the substances in this last category can be lifesaving, bacteria are able to outsmart them quickly, and they should be reserved for appropriate use.

Now let's move on to chapter 3 for some self-care strategies and alternative therapies that can help to resolve common illnesses *before* you need to call the doctor.

3

PROTECTING YOUR HEALTH

Today, more than ever, you must be your own health bodyguard. You must make informed choices regarding the prevention and treatment of illness to keep yourself and your family healthy. Gone are the days when doctors made house calls and knew your entire family's health history—if those days ever existed. In our transient society, where career changes or corporate transfers may require you to move frequently, the doctor you trust today may not be the one you see tomorrow.

An Ounce of Prevention

Since the turn of the last century, our nation has focused much of its scientific resources on treating diseases, using the best medical interventions available. While treating disease is critical, especially in the early stages when treatment works best, there is a compelling case supported by a host of scientific data that the prevention of illness should be our utmost goal. We can actually make a difference in staying healthy—if we make the effort to change negative lifestyle habits and take some other preventive measures.

According to the U.S. Department of Health and Human Services and the Centers for Disease Control and Prevention (CDC), $1 spent on diabetes education saves from $2 to $3 in hospitalization costs; the cost of preventing one cavity through water fluoridation is about $4 (compare that with the cost of filling a cavity!); and people who participate in an arthritis self-help course may save $267 in health care costs over 4 years—and experience less pain and greater mobility. Other statistics suggest that preventive measures such as health screening, immunization, and individual lifestyle changes could eliminate an estimated 23 percent of premature cancer deaths, more than 50 percent of the serious complications of diabetes, and 45 percent of the premature deaths from cardiovascular diseases.

Given that preventing illness is such a smart move for both your body and your wallet, it is hard to believe how few people are willing to do what it takes to stay well. As a health-risk analyst, I know that taking control of such habits as a high-fat diet, a sedentary lifestyle, the use of tobacco and drugs, and the abuse of alcohol could prevent between 40 and 70 percent of all premature deaths, a third of all cases of acute disability, and two-thirds of all cases of chronic disability. I also know that disease prevention is a surefire way to avoid overkill.

Your Body's Natural Defenses

The most effective way to stay well is to keep your immune system strong. If you take care of yourself with a nutritious diet high in phytochemicals (naturally occurring chemical substances in plants, such as an-

The Antioxidant Success Story

Most doctors endorse the role of antioxidants in fighting disease, including one in the *Journal of the American College of Nutrition.* Studies have found that antioxidants protect the body from the formation of *free radicals*—atoms or groups of atoms that can damage cells, weaken the immune system, and lead to infection and degenerative diseases like cancer and heart disease. To boost your immune function and aid your body in healing, make sure your diet includes plenty of foods rich in these antioxidants:

Beta-carotene. Found in apricots, broccoli, cantaloupes, carrots, collard greens, papayas, peaches, pumpkins, spinach, sweet potatoes, and tomatoes, beta-carotene is converted to vitamin A in the body.

Selenium. This trace mineral helps to protect your cells against toxins and is critical to immune function. Good food sources include Brazil nuts, meats, poultry, and seafood.

Vitamin C. Whole-food sources of vitamin C include broccoli, cantaloupes, citrus fruits, kiwifruit, peppers, potatoes, strawberries, tomatoes, and blueberries.

Vitamin E. Vitamin E is important for the maintenance of cell membranes. This vitamin is found in wheat germ, nuts and seeds, margarine, and whole grains.

tioxidants, that help to prevent cell damage), plenty of physical exercise, healing sleep, and a minimum of stress, you can stay well and avoid chronic illness to a remarkable degree.

The main function of your immune system is to distinguish "self" (your bodily system) from "non-self" (invading germs) through a complex network of antibodies, proteins, and specialized cells. All of these have a mission, which is to keep you healthy by attacking and destroying foreign materials. When your receptor cells sense trouble, they signal to the antibodies and other cells to stop the *antigens*, which are the invading bacteria, viruses, parasites, or fungi. When some part of this process fails, the immune system itself fails to function as it should, and you get sick.

When to Take Antibiotics—And When to Refrain

Besides eating right, getting enough sleep and exercise, and avoiding stress, another key way to keep your immune system healthy over the long term is to use antibiotics only when they are necessary. When bacteria are repeatedly exposed to antibiotics, such as when you take the medication needlessly or too frequently, the germs in your body change. These changes can make the germs stronger than before so they fight the antibiotic—and win. Once your immune system becomes compromised, your illness may linger with no signs of improvement or it may suddenly take a turn for the worse, requiring you to seek emergency medical care. In addition, those around you may get the resistant bacteria and come down with a similar illness that is very difficult to treat.

The same caution applies to other types of drugs, including antifungal or antiparasitic agents. Just as you wouldn't take aspirin for an upset stomach or an antidiarrhea medicine for a yeast infection, don't take an antibiotic unless it is indicated for the ailment and prescribed by your doctor. Certainly, do not root in your medicine cabinet for unfinished antibiotics from a previous illness, thinking that these will cure you. If you get to the point of thinking you need antibiotics, this means that you should talk—and listen—to your doctor.

When your doctor says "no antibiotics needed" for a cold or flu, that's the truth. *Antibiotics only work against bacterial infections*. They do not work against viral infections, and viruses cause most colds, flu, and sore throats. If your cold develops into a secondary infection, such as bacterial bronchitis or ear infection, then your doctor may recommend and prescribe an antibiotic. If you have a chronic illness or impaired immune function,

Taking Antibiotics Responsibly

- When you see your doctor, do not demand antibiotics. Your doctor will try to determine whether you have a bacterial infection or a virus and will prescribe antibiotics only if necessary.
- If your doctor prescribes antibiotics, don't be afraid to use them. While your body may develop resistant bacteria when you take antibiotics, after you finish your course of treatment, the nonresistant bacteria will return and compete with the resistant ones. As a result, the resistant bacteria may not exist in sufficient numbers to lead to illness.
- Use antibiotics exactly as prescribed. Take the full course of treatment on time and as directed, and do not save pills "just in case" you might get sick later on.
- Do not give your antibiotics to anyone else, and do not take someone else's medication.

your doctor may consider an antibiotic earlier on in an illness, but unless your doctor specifically instructs you otherwise, save the antibiotics for severe infections. The sooner we all take responsibility for our health and the appropriate use of antibiotics, the longer we will be able to have antibiotics play their critical role in our pharmaceutical arsenal.

America's Love Affair with Medicine

Statistics show that of all health care costs, the fastest growing segment is pharmaceuticals—a direct result of the Age of Miracles. The cost of outpatient prescription drugs rose from $12 billion in 1980 to a stunning $55.5 billion in 1995 to $145 billion in 2000, according to a report released in 2001 by the pharmaceutical market research firm IMS Health. Of course, many of these drugs are being used successfully and appropriately to cure or manage an illness. No one is questioning the necessity of insulin for diabetes, chemotherapy for cancer, or antibiotics for bacterial infections. But some drugs are taken unnecessarily because we have neglected to live and react to illness responsibly.

Just by watching television you are introduced to the latest pharmaceutical treatment for every kind of ailment from depression, PMS, and obesity to urinary incontinence, nasal congestion, and impotence. And you don't even have to seek a medical diagnosis, as most so-called lifestyle medications are available for purchase on the Internet if not over-the-counter at your local pharmacy. While you should never forego a medication that you really need, it is important to be sure that you really need any medications that you take because all medications, including antibiotics, can have side effects. Remember that antibiotics cure only certain bacteria-related illnesses; if taken carelessly, you may get more serious health problems than you bargained for.

Should We Blame the Media?

Some people would like to blame our overuse of antibiotics on media campaigns that now market directly to consumers. There are ads for even strong prescription drugs, including antibiotics, as pharmaceutical companies work hard to ensure that consumers are aware of their products. It's true that drug advertising has more than tripled in dollar volume, from $791 million in 1996 to $2.5 billion in 2000. But the media are no more to blame than consumers who are still wrapped up in the Age of Miracles and have not yet embraced the Age of Risk Management. As one physician shared, "A patient may come to my office on Friday with a sore throat and demand that I give her antibiotics. When I don't give her an antibiotic but tell her to increase her intake of liquids, get more rest, and take an analgesic, she leaves unconvinced, thinking I'm not a qualified physician. The next week she shops around for another doctor and tells all her friends to do the same."

Unfortunately, this demand for a quick fix has fueled our resistance crisis. In 1954, 2 million pounds of antibiotics were produced in the United States. Today, that figure exceeds 50 million pounds, according to a study in *Medical Clinics of North America* in 2001. Also, a 1998 Institute of Medicine report estimated the extent of the problem, that antibiotic resistance costs as much as $30 *billion* annually in the United States alone, as doctors must search for more powerful and expensive drugs to stop bacterial infections.

Without a doubt, antibiotics are lifesaving drugs. But when you learn that more than 12 million antibiotic prescriptions were given in 1992 to adults in the United States for upper respiratory tract infections and bronchitis, on which these drugs may have little or no effect, you have to be concerned. Another $500 million worth of antibiotics are prescribed annually just for ear infections in children—which, in many cases, may not require antibiotic therapy. The same is true for sore throats. In a revealing study published in 1999 in the *British Medical Journal*, 716 people, age 4 and older, with sore throats were split into three groups. One group was given antibiotics, while one group received no treatment at all. The third group of volunteers was given antibiotics if the symptoms continued for more than 3 days. More than a third of the patients in each group reported feeling better by the third day, and through the duration of the illness, the number of days off work or school and the number of patients who were satisfied with their treatment was essentially the same. More and more studies are concluding the same thing: that antibiotics are *not* necessary for curing many common illnesses.

Treating the Body, Mind, and Spirit

If antibiotics are not the miracle cure we once thought, then where should you turn for treatment? With the soaring costs of health care, many consumers are turning to alternative therapies for self-care and treatment. This school of *complementary* or *alternative* medicine views the mind and body as an integrated system—meaning they influence each other—and counts on your commitment to staying well.

In the past three decades, alternative medicine has soared in popularity and now touts a wide range of nonstandard approaches to personal health and healing. While conventional medical doctors focus on defining disease based on measurable symptoms and then eliminating them and any underlying cause of disease, alternative therapy practitioners focus on treating the whole person—body, mind, and spirit—with the focus on staying balanced and well. Alternative remedies, which range from herbal or vitamin supplements to mind/body exercises, are generally safe, relatively affordable, and easily accessible.

But is alternative medicine really a radical new prescription? Here is where we must first take a clue from those in the know—scientists and conventional medical doctors who express caution, as most alternative treatments have not passed clinical trials. No matter what the advertising flyer claims at the natural foods store, even the most popular medicinal herbs with pharmaceutical compounds have ingredients that have not been tested and are not scrutinized by the Food and Drug Administration (FDA). Unlike products that have FDA approval, herbal products have not gone through a clinical trial to show that they are safe and effective before going on to the market.

Nonetheless, a growing body of scientists and medical doctors are advocating alternative therapies as safe with no substantiated harmful side

About Immune-Enhancing Herbs

Keep in mind that herbs that bolster your immune function act as antibiotics—over time, you build up a tolerance to their therapeutic effects, and their efficacy wears off after continuous use. It is best to rotate use of immune-supporting herbs. Be moderate and safe with these healing herbs, and note the following warnings when using certain herbs:

Echinacea (*Echinacea purpurea* or *E. angustifolia*): This commonly ingested herb can cause allergic reactions in some people. It is not recommended for those with autoimmune disorders such as lupus because echinacea boosts the immune system's activity, and autoimmune diseases are caused by an overactive immune system.

Garlic (*Allium sativum*): Garlic is actually a medicinal herb. Avoid it if you are contemplating surgery because large amounts can reduce blood-clotting time. For the same reason, garlic can also be dangerous for people taking blood-thinning drugs such as warfarin (Coumadin).

Goldenseal (*Hydrastis canadensis*): People with hypoglycemia, children, and the elderly should not take goldenseal without a physician's guidance. It is not recommended for long-term use.

effects, noting that these may be considered along with your scientifically proven conventional treatments. As we learn more about them, some alternative therapies may emerge as the best strategies, while others may emerge as ones that could lead to severe side effects. Although a great deal of uncertainty surrounds these approaches because they have not been tested as rigorously as traditional medicines, this does *not* mean that they do not work. You should also appreciate that any treatment may work differently for some people than for others. You need to pay attention to what works for you!

Use Alternative with Conventional Therapies

In this book, I have tried to cover the wealth of options that you might have when suffering from an illness and to take a positive move toward unifying the conventional with the alternative, while respecting your health care preferences. Yet, there are some stumbling blocks. For ex-

Seek Professional Advice

The Dietary Supplement Health and Education Act of 1994 states that the Food and Drug Administration (FDA) has no legal authority to require companies to prove that their products are effective or safe, nor can it enforce quality standards. In fact, for dietary supplements and ethnic remedies, the FDA must demonstrate that a product is harmful before it can remove it from the market. This contrasts dramatically with the criteria for pharmaceutical drugs, which must be tested for safety and efficacy before they go on the market. Most supplements can be made and sold as snake oil was years ago, which means only one thing: *You are not protected.* It is your right as a consumer to know that supplements are not regulated as to their claims or their potencies. In other words, there are no laws requiring these products to do what they claim to do or even that the ingredients are what the label says they are.

Therefore, it's smart to consult a trusted health professional to help you determine the right remedies to try, to advise you in selecting these products, and to warn you about possible interactions with prescription drugs or over-the-counter medications. Follow the dosage from your health care provider and on the label carefully. (Also, since plants can vary significantly in their potency, the chances are greater that you will get what you pay for if you buy a brand labeled "standardized.") Most important, keep a record of what you take, how much, and when, so if complications arise you will be able to provide this information to your doctor and other people who are helping you. For more information on herbal therapies, see the References section, starting on page 318.

ample, one of the most common mistakes made by some people when they use alternative medicine practitioners is that they stop the traditional medical treatment altogether, and sometimes a supplement or herb may counteract the effects of your prescription medication. Both situations leave your doctor baffled when the medicine is ineffective and your illness worsens.

As a rule of thumb, when our immune systems falter and we battle the resulting ailments such as frequent colds, sore throats, skin problems, allergies, backaches, and ulcers, alternative therapies may help to resolve these problems, especially if we focus on changing lifestyle habits, apply self-care early on, and practice preventive measures to stay well. But serious medical treatments such as fixing a broken bone, treating bacterial pneumonia, running a blood glucose test or colon cancer screening, or checking out an unusual lump or bleeding mole clearly falls within the arena of your conventional medical doctor. Your preferences for the mode of health care you pursue are important, and I will respect them as I tell you how to use what you learned in chapter 2 about your personal health risks and your Risk Quotient (RQ) in dealing with some common illnesses.

Let Your RQ Guide You to Good Health

For the remainder of this chapter, I have identified 31 common illnesses that are treated—and mistreated—with antibiotics. These conditions afflict adults, causing loss of workdays, reduced income, and poor quality of life. Since I am not a doctor of medicine, I am not qualified to give you medical advice; and even though several doctors reviewed parts of this book, you should consult your physician about any medical treatment.

(continued on page 80)

About the Remedies in This Chapter

Read the instructions on all herbal and supplemental remedies before using them. Some remedies should not be used by pregnant or lactating women; consult your doctor before taking any herbal or nutritional remedy. Never discontinue any prescription medication without first talking to your doctor, and consider the following:

Acetaminophen (Tylenol). If you have or are at risk for renal and/or liver failure, always consult your physician before taking acetaminophen.

Acidophilus (*Lactobacillus acidophilus*). If you have any serious gastrointestinal problems that require medical attention, check with your doctor before supplementing. If you are taking antibiotics, take them at least 2 hours before supplementing.

Astragalus (*Astragalus membranaceus*). Astragalus may cause loose stools or abdominal bloating.

Comfrey (*Symphytum officinale*). Do not ingest comfrey or apply it to deep, gaping, or infected wounds, as it is potentially toxic in those situations.

Echinacea (*Echinacea purpurea* or *E. angustifolia*). Do not use if you are allergic to closely related plants such as ragweed, asters, and chrysanthemums. Since echinacea stimulates the immune system, do not use if you have tuberculosis or an autoimmune condition such as lupus or multiple sclerosis. Use echinacea for up to 8 weeks.

Folic acid. Use folic acid only for a few days, as long-term use can deplete vitamin B12.

Ginkgo (*Ginkgo biloba*). Do not take ginkgo with MAO inhibitors, aspirin, or nonsteroidal anti-inflammatory drugs (NSAIDs) such as ibuprofen. Use with caution if you're already taking warfarin (Coumadin).

Goldenseal (*Hydrastis canadensis*). Do not take goldenseal if you have pollen allergies or high blood pressure, and only take it for 2 to 3 weeks.

Ibuprofen (Advil). Always take ibuprofen and other NSAIDs with food. If you have or are at risk for renal and/or liver failure, always consult your physician before taking ibuprofen. Avoid ibuprofen if you are allergic to aspirin, as it may cause wheezing and congestion.

Licorice (*Glycyrrhiza glabra*). Do not ingest licorice if you have high blood pressure, diabetes, liver or kidney disorders, or low potassium levels. Do not use for more than 6 weeks.

Papain (papaya enzyme). If you have allergies to pollen, talk to your doctor before taking papaya enzyme tablets.

Uva-ursi (*Arctostaphylos uva-ursi*). Do not take uva-ursi for longer than 2 weeks, and do not use if you have kidney disease.

Vitamin A. Because vitamin A is not water soluble, do not exceed safe levels if you supplement; it can reach toxic levels.

Vitamin C (ascorbic acid). Don't supplement with vitamin C if you are prone to kidney stones; talk to your doctor.

Vitamin E. If you take vitamin E supplements, be sure to use top-quality vitamin E, either the d-alpha or mixed tocopherol types (not synthetic d,l-alpha vitamin E).

Water. If you are taking prescription diuretics or your doctor has advised you to limit your fluid intake, do not increase your water intake without first checking with your doctor.

Zinc. Avoid taking too much zinc in supplement form because it is toxic in high doses. Zinc may cause nausea; to avoid this side effect with lozenges, suck on them after a meal or snack.

Recognizing that many people may want to pursue alternative medicine approaches, however, I have chosen to include the recommendations of a widely published naturopathic physician, Chris D. Meletis, N.D., dean of naturopathic medicine and chief medical officer at the National College of Naturopathic Medicine in Portland, Oregon. Dr. Meletis has outlined some excellent preventive measures and alternative remedies you can use at home, depending on your Risk Quotient. Even if these common ailments are not a problem at this time, you can still boost your immune function to help avoid serious illness and reduce the need for antibiotics later on.

The lists on the following pages cover only some of the possibilities for self-care, and there may be many more natural remedies that may help. It's important to consider these suggestions as a beginning, and to consult with your health care provider, as you become empowered to look for safe strategies to stay well. You will also need to consult with a qualified provider to obtain instructions for using any therapies, and you should always carefully follow the directions on the label of any product—both herbal and conventional—that you use. Pregnant or lactating women should consult their doctors before taking any herbal or nutritional remedy. Seek medical advice before you stop taking any prescription medicine, whether this is prescription diuretics, antibiotics, or other medicines. See "Dietary Reference Intakes" on page 164 for more information on safe supplement levels, and see "About the Remedies in This Chapter" on pages 78 and 79 for cautions and things to consider when using both herbal and supplemental remedies.

Risk Quotients 1 through 4

If you are basically healthy and scored in RQs 1 through 4 in the Personal Health Risk Profile, then alternative therapies may play a successful role in helping you prevent and even end an acute or chronic illness such as sinusitis, bronchitis, or gastrointestinal distress, among many others. The suggestions offered for each RQ are designed to build up, so you should read and consider all the suggestions for each RQ up to the level of your Risk Quotient. For example, if you are RQ 4, consider the self-care suggestions in RQs 1, 2, and 3 before using the tips in RQ 4. Again, do not close the door on traditional therapies for serious illness, and always recognize your doctor's important role in your overall health program. Also keep in mind that any preexisting conditions and allergies should factor in to your self-care decisions.

Risk Quotient 5

If you have a compromised immune system, chronic illness, or scored a 5 for your Risk Quotient, work with your doctor. Your conventional medical doctor is someone you must trust to run the necessary tests, make an accurate diagnosis, and give you quick and effective medical treatment to stop infections and keep you well, including prescribing antibiotics if necessary. Even so, following the basic prevention strategies provided for Risk Quotients 1 through 4 may improve your health and significantly lower your risk of overkill, and you should discuss these with your doctor.

Abscess

What Is It? Fairly common among adults of all ages, an abscess is a localized collection of pus and infection on or in the skin or below the skin (subcutaneous tissue). Using self-care remedies early on may help you avoid antibiotic therapy or an invasive procedure to open the abscess.

What Causes It? An abscess can occur anywhere on the body. Sometimes an abscess occurs after a bacterial infection (*Staphylococcus aureus* is a common cause) at the site of a cut or abrasion, as a complication of boils (carbuncles or furuncles), or an infected hair follicle (folliculitis). The degree of seriousness largely depends upon location of infection as well as the size of the abscess.

Signs and Symptoms: An open wound or abrasion becomes inflamed, swollen, and reddened and starts to drain fluid. The skin lesion is tender and warm to the touch as the abscess worsens.

Prevention and Treatment:

RQ 1 **Apply moist heat.** Frequently use a warm moist compress to enhance circulation, bringing white blood cells and oxygen to the area and helping to encourage the abscess to drain. Removing the offending agent by drainage is the key to reducing inflammation and pain. By increasing blood flow to the wound, heat helps to speed healing.

Try a poultice. A poultice—a moist herbal preparation spread onto the affected area of the body and covered with a clean, dry cloth—can help. Some people find that a neutral temperature, betonite clay poultice has a drawing effect on abscesses. (To avoid damaging the skin, make sure the tissue is not too sensitive.) Add fresh or dried comfrey (*Symphytum officinale*) to the poultice. Comfrey is an herb that contains allantoin, which promotes new cell growth. You can find betonite clay and comfrey at most natural foods stores.

RQ 2 **Boost your intake of vitamin C.** Eat whole foods high in vitamin C, and consider taking a supplement to boost your intake of this important antioxidant. (See "Dietary Reference Intakes" on page 164.) Vitamin C is considered essential for the health of collagen, a component of the skin, and also protects against infection and aids in wound health. Foods high in vitamin C include broccoli, oranges, peppers, cantaloupes, strawberries, grapefruit, tomatoes, and kiwifruit.

Cut out sweets. Sugar may fuel bacterial growth and inhibit immune function, so lower your sugar intake and favor sugar-free foods. Also check labels for corn sweetener, corn syrup, malted barley, molasses, fructose, dextrose, and sucrose, which are other names for sugar.

RQ 3 **Take a healing herbal combo.** Try the herbs echinacea (*Echinacea purpurea* or *E. angustifolia*) and goldenseal (*Hydrastis canadensis*)—readily available at drug stores, natural foods stores, and even supermarkets. Both are said to have antimicrobial and anti-inflammatory effects in the body. Echinacea may help fight both viral and bacterial infections, although how it does this is not yet fully understood.

Eat more fresh garlic. Garlic (*Allium sativum*) has both antimicrobial and immunostimulating properties. It also releases a powerful antibiotic called allicin. Garlic was used for medicinal purposes by the Greeks, Romans, and Egyptians.

RQ 4 **Apply tea tree oil.** To feel relief and speed natural healing, combine 1 part tea tree oil (*Melaleuca alternifolia*) with 4 parts olive oil and apply externally to the affected area 3 to 4 times daily. Do not apply to exceptionally sensitive skin, around eyes, or near mucous membranes, and discontinue if irritation occurs. Tea tree oil is available at most natural foods stores.

Use a paste. Open a capsule of dried goldenseal (*Hydrastis canadensis*) and mix it with water to make a paste; then apply it to the affected area. Do not use goldenseal once the boil has ruptured since this herb can cause permanent staining of the skin as the wound heals.

Think zinc! Zinc is vital to the body's resistance to infection and for tissue repair. While a vitamin-mineral supplement with zinc can boost your intake of this mineral, you should also include whole foods high in zinc—oysters, shellfish, eggs, lean red meat, lean pork, chicken, turkey, fortified cereals, baked beans, low-fat milk and yogurt, and tofu—in your diet.

When to Call the Doctor: Treated early, skin abscesses are rarely a problem and should improve in a few days. However, if the infection continues untreated or if your immune system is compromised, the abscess may obstruct the functioning of deeper body tissues, which may result in the infection spreading locally or systemically in the bloodstream and possibly affecting the entire body. If you have signs of worsening infection such as fever, pain, redness, localized swelling, and drainage that looks like pus or is bloody, call your doctor immediately. Also, a gum abscess or suspected internal (body cavity) abscess should be immediately assessed by your physician.

Your doctor will diagnose an abscess by physical examination and appearance. In some cases, a culture is taken of the drainage to see which bacteria are causing the infection. Your doctor may have to lance and clean the abscessed area, removing pus and infected material to stop the infection.

Acne

What Is It? Acne is an inflammatory skin problem that typically appears on the face, scalp, neck, shoulders, chest, and back and is characterized by clogged pores, tender pimples, and irritated skin. Starting at puberty, it's estimated that three out of four teenagers have acne. But acne is not just for kids! This skin disease can continue into adulthood, affecting men and women alike.

One of the many functions of skin, the body's largest organ, is to help detoxify your body. It's not surprising that your body's internal health is often reflected in the skin's quality and tone. While extreme cases of acne can cause pitting and scarring of the skin, if you treat the condition quickly, it is rarely this serious.

What Causes It? It's thought that acne is caused by hormonal changes that stimulate the oil-producing (sebaceous) skin glands. Other hormonal changes including pregnancy, menstrual periods, and the use of birth control pills can aggravate acne for some women (although in other women, birth control pills can improve acne or have no effect). Even stress is a known trigger. If effective prevention and treatment measures are started early, you can manage acne and keep it under control.

Signs and Symptoms: Acne starts when blocked pores on the skin produce a *whitehead.* If the pore begins to trap dirt, the top surface of the plug may darken, resulting in a *blackhead.* When the blocked pores become infected or inflamed, it causes a *pimple* or raised red spot with a white center. *Cysts* form when the blockage and inflammation deep inside hair follicles produce lumps beneath the surface of the skin.

Prevention and Treatment:

RQ 1 **Keep your face clean.** Acne treatments work by reducing oil production, speeding up skin cell turnover, fighting bacterial infection, or doing all three. Start by washing problem areas with a gentle cleanser and warm water two or three times a day. Avoid overwashing, as this causes irritation. Also avoid picking or popping the pimples.

Shun facial irritants. Avoid facial scrubs, scented soaps, and astringents, as they may cause irritation of the skin, leading to a new breakout of acne. Apply over-the-counter acne medications with benzoyl peroxide.

RQ 2 **Eliminate the offenders.** Avoid certain foods such as alcohol, caffeine (affects liver detoxification), hydrogenated oils, fried food, and cigarette smoking. While these do not cause the problem, they may work to trigger or worsen acne.

Stay regular. Make sure you have regular bowel movements so that toxins are properly eliminated. A high-fiber diet high in complex carbohydrates (fruits, vegetables, and whole grains) can help to eliminate toxins.

Drink H_2O. Staying hydrated with plenty of water intake throughout the day is important to detoxify the body, helping to eliminate impurities.

Add Vitamin E. Vitamin E is a powerful antioxidant important for the maintenance of cell membranes. Some studies, including one in the *Journal of Nutrition*, reveal that vitamin E helps to stimulate the function of T-cells, which are important fighters of the immune system. Vitamin E-rich foods include almonds, lobster, corn oil, cod-liver oil, safflower oil, salmon steak, hazelnuts, and sunflower seeds.

RQ 3 **Add other supplements.** Take zinc, vitamin C, and essential fatty acids (EFAs). (See "Dietary Reference Intakes" on page 164.) Zinc helps to fight infection, boost immune function, promote wound healing, and aid hormone metabolism. Vitamin C helps ensure proper collagen formation and skin integrity. EFAs are not manufactured by the body but are essential to good health and are available in fish and flaxseed oils, which contain omega-3.

How to De-Stress

If you need to de-stress, try soothing music. A study done at Saint Agnes Hospital in Baltimore found that when patients in critical care units listened to half an hour of classical music, the listening had the same effect as antianxiety medications.

"B" calm. Because stress is thought to trigger some acne breakouts, take a vitamin B complex. Revealing studies have shown that by including plenty of foods high in complex carbohydrates in your diet, you can boost the level of serotonin, a naturally occurring neurotransmitter that has a calming influence on the body. Foods that are rich in tryptophan, along with vitamin B_6, provide the building blocks your body needs to make serotonin. Tryptophan-rich foods include brown rice, cottage cheese, lean meat, and soy protein.

RQ 4 **Take vitamin A.** Eat whole foods high in vitamin A, a powerful antioxidant that has been shown to boost healing in problem skin as well as protect the skin from the damaging effects of the sun's ultraviolet rays. Foods high in beta-carotene, a critical building block your body needs to make vitamin A, include carrots, sweet potatoes, apricots, cantaloupes, pumpkins, pink grapefruit, tomatoes, peaches, and collard greens. (But be careful because although beta-carotene does not build up in your system, vitamin A can.)

Use herbal therapies. Goldenseal (*Hydrastis canadensis*), echinacea (*Echinacea purpurea* or *E. angustifolia*), and garlic (*Allium sativum*) can bolster immune function and help combat infection. These herbs are available at most grocery or natural foods stores.

Use natural healing. A poultice—a moist herbal preparation spread onto the affected area of the body and covered with a clean, dry cloth—can help. Apply a poultice made of 1 part apple cider vinegar and 10 parts filtered water to the affected area. Keep this away from eyes and other sensitive tissues, as it may burn.

Chill! Stress wreaks havoc with hormones and may lower your immune defenses. Learn how to work periods of time-out or relaxation into your daily routine to ease tension and give your body time to recover. Stand up and stretch or take a walk.

When to Call the Doctor: While acne is not a serious medical condition, you may want to seek medical treatment from a dermatologist for persistent pimples or inflamed cysts to avoid scarring or other damage to your skin. If acne or the scars it may have left are affecting your social relationships or self-esteem, you may also want to see a dermatologist to see whether your acne can be controlled or scars can be diminished. In rare cases, a sudden onset of severe acne in an adult may signal an underlying disease such as the hormonal disorder polycystic ovarian syndrome (PCOS), a leading cause of infertility. If acne strikes suddenly or without explanation, see your doctor.

Bedsores

What Is It? Bedsores, or decubitus ulcers, are potentially serious wounds that occur in people who are either bedridden or confined to a chair. Usually found in the sacral area (lower back), bed sores also occur on the hips, shoulders, elbows, ears, back of the head, and ankles. The only way for bedsores to fully heal is to control or manage the underlying cause.

What Causes It? Prolonged pressure on a bony part of the body (e.g., an elbow) causes bedsores. When you are bedridden for days or weeks, pressure in the same location irritates the skin, causing the wound to form.

Signs and Symptoms: A bedsore starts out as irritated or chafed skin. It may be warm, pink, or even red before the skin breaks. In time, the skin forms a small blister or crater. In later stages of bedsores, the wound deepens into the layer of fat beneath the skin. It may be white or black in color and drain a foul-smelling liquid. Bedsores are extremely serious when the muscle or bone is seen in the deepest part of the wound.

Prevention and Treatment:

RQ 1 **Avoid problems.** Bedsores may or may not get infected, but it's best to avoid them altogether. You can do this by repositioning your body every 1 or 2 hours during the day if you are bedridden or confined to a chair. If you are in bed and comfortable in most positions, it is good to lie on one side, then your back, then the other side. Also keep sheets and bedding stretched flat to avoid bunching and wrinkles, which can irritate skin.

Cushion the pressure points. Place pillows at strategic points on your body (under the heels, elbows, and between the knees) to protect the common pressure points. Also make sure that the clothing you wear is smooth with no seams or buttons that can irritate one place on your body. Maintain good circulation by sitting up or walking around periodically, if you are able.

RQ 2 **Heal the wound.** Use calendula (*Calendula officinalis*) ointment, found at most natural foods stores, to help with the healing of superficial wounds. Calendula is a flower that has been known for centuries as a natural healing and soothing substance when applied locally. (An ointment usually is made with a petroleum derivative that adds moisture to the skin, so use with caution if your skin is oily. A gel is less greasy and does not clog pores as readily.)

Up your essential fatty acids. Supplements of essential fatty acids (EFAs), such as cold pressed fish oil or cod-liver oil, flaxseed oil, evening primrose oil (*Oenothera biennis*), black currant oil (*Ribes* *nigrum*), or borage oil (*Borago officinalis*) can help to boost immune function, enhance overall skin health and integrity, and reduce inflammation since EFAs are not manufactured by the body. All of these oils can be found at most grocery and natural foods stores; store them in a cool, dark place.

RQ 3 **Eat your weedies.** A well-balanced diet of fresh fruits and vegetables can help to maintain immune function. Be sure you have sufficient protein and caloric intake, as well. (An average adult needs 45 to 55 grams of protein each day.)

Try an herbal cocktail. Supplementing with the immune-boosting herbs echinacea (*Echinacea purpurea* or *E. angustifolia*) and garlic (*Allium sativum*) may help your bedsores to heal quickly. Echinacea is thought by some to fight bacterial and viral infections, while garlic is a known antimicrobial—important so the sore does not worsen.

RQ 4 **Use a healing oil.** The oil from a vitamin E capsule may help to speed healing when directly applied on the superficial wound. Vitamin E may also improve the effect of wound dressings on large scars. Use either the oil-filled capsules or pure vitamin E oil found at most grocery or natural foods stores.

Add herbal therapy. Take goldenseal (*Hydrastis canadensis*), a known antibacterial, and ginkgo (*Ginkgo biloba*), which aids circulation, to help bedsores heal.

Lighten up. Use an egg crate mattress or air mattress to help lighten and distribute your body weight.

When to Call the Doctor: Bedsores in the early stage can be managed with alternative therapies and alternating positions. But if the sore worsens and turns black, has a foul-smelling drainage, or if there are signs the muscle or bone may be exposed, seek emergency care.

Bites and Stings

What Is It? Insect bites and stings are tiny wounds in the skin caused by a variety of biting or stinging insects such as mosquitoes, wasps, gnats, horseflies, fleas, or chiggers.

What Causes It? When the insect bites and injects venom or other foreign agent into your skin, this triggers an allergic (immune) reaction.

Signs and Symptoms: After being bitten or stung, you may notice localized swelling of the skin that may last a few hours or days before fading away. Sometimes an insect bite or sting will cause an itchy pinkish rash. Bites and stings can burn or throb if there is a great deal of swelling. If the wound becomes infected, you may notice that it is red, swollen, warm to touch, and has a puslike drainage.

Prevention and Treatment: In all cases, clean the area with rubbing alcohol, taking care so the stinger is not pushed into the skin even further—but don't delay removing any stinger if rubbing alcohol isn't available. For bee stings, scrape off the stinger with a blade or fingernail, but do not remove it with tweezers, which may squeeze more venom out of the venom sac. In contrast, always remove ticks using tweezers because this increases the chance of removing the tick's mouthparts, which, if left in the skin, can cause persistent irritation. Also be very careful to avoid rupturing the tick, and wear gloves if you can while removing the tick to avoid contamination with tick fluids that may be infected.

RQ 1 **Prevent bites.** Wear clothing that protects the body, apply insect repellent, burn citronella (*Cymbopogon nardus*) candles, avoid heavy perfumes or fragrances, keep doors and windows closed or screened, and make sure your pets keep free of insects.

Use kitchen-cabinet cures. Cover the sting with a paste made of water mixed with meat tenderizer that contains either bromelain (pineapple extract) or papain (papaya extract). You can also simply cover the sting with a slice of papaya. Some people find that a paste made out of baking soda and water can also be helpful.

Ice it. After you've applied the paste, cover the bite with an ice pack. The ice compress will help prevent the spread of the venom.

RQ 2 **Stop the allergic reaction.** Bee stings cause allergic reactions in nearly 1 out of 100 people, with reaction symptoms ranging from numb lips to severe anaphylactic shock. Try to stop the allergic reaction by supplementing with vitamin C, a natural antihistamine, and quercetin, a highly potent bioflavonoid (a natural plant chemical) found in citrus fruits, red and yellow onions, and broccoli. Both of these antioxidants reduce inflammation by lessening the production of histamine, a substance produced by the body that causes the allergic reaction on the skin (or on other parts of the body).

RQ 3 **Reduce the swelling.** Take Benadryl, an over-the-counter antihistamine, to stop swelling. If the swelling continues, call your doctor to make sure you are not allergic to the sting.

Try homeopathy. *Apis mellifica*, a homeopathic therapy, may reduce the symptoms of inflammation and allergic reactions. This remedy is available at natural foods stores.

Boost immune function. Take the herbs echinacea (*Echinacea purpurea* or *E. angustifolia*) and goldenseal (*Hydrastis canadensis*) to bolster your immune function and help speed wound healing.

RQ 4 **Keep a watchful eye.** Even after using the self-care tips in Risk Quotients 1 through 3, you need to keep a watchful eye on the sting or bite if your Risk Quotient is 4. Normally, a sting or bite should not get infected, but if you notice an abscess or pus pocket forming and the offending insect is not known, call your doctor. Certain creatures, such as spiders and scorpions, can cause tissue necrosis (death) that can be severe.

When to Call the Doctor: Most bites and stings do not require emergency care, but if you are one of the two million Americans who are allergic to insect stings, you could have an allergic reaction, including anaphylactic shock, and may need immediate medical intervention. Watch for symptoms of hoarseness, difficulty swallowing, trouble breathing, severe swelling, and other systemic effects beyond the local sting or bite area. If your ear lobes, tongue, lips, or eyes swell, or if you have stomach cramps, seek urgent medical care. Antihistamines, steroids, or epinephrine (adrenaline) may be needed to reduce swelling.

Bladder Infections (Cystitis)

What Is It? Infection of the bladder is common in more women than men because the female urethra is shorter and closer to the anus.

What Causes It? Most bladder infections begin in the urinary tract (see "Urinary Tract Infections," page 158)—if left untreated, the infection progresses to the bladder—and are caused by *E. coli*, a bacterium that is normally found in your intestine. Under perfect conditions, the urethra and bladder excrete "bad" bacteria during urination.

Signs and Symptoms: When bacteria remain in the bladder, they can multiply quickly and result in infection with symptoms such as pressure in the lower pelvis, painful and frequent urination, cloudy urine, blood in urine, and a strong urine odor.

Prevention and Treatment:

RQ 1 **Use the rules of good hygiene.** Women can dramatically decrease their risk of bladder infections by wiping from front to back after going to the bathroom.

Stay hydrated. Drink 8 glasses (64 ounces) of water daily to help the urine stay diluted and to encourage kidney function.

Urinate frequently. Urinating frequently throughout the day helps to prevent urine from becoming stagnant. Go immediately after intercourse to avoid "honeymoon cystitis."

Stay moist. Make sure vaginal tissues stay moist and avoid irritation that could cause swelling, making it difficult to urinate.

Eliminate diuretics. To reduce pain and irritation, try eliminating caffeine and other diuretics that can be dehydrating.

RQ 2 **Drink unsweetened cranberry juice.** Cranberry juice contains arbutin, a chemical compound that is antibiotic. Some studies show that cranberry juice lowers *E. coli* adhesion to bladder walls, while other juices such as orange or grapefruit do not. Drinking 17 ounces (a little more than 2 cups) of cranberry juice daily is recommended to treat a bladder infection, or take cranberry (*Vaccinium macrocarpon*) concentrate capsules and drink 8 glasses of water each day. To prevent bladder infection, try 1 glass of juice daily.

Avoid sugar. Eating too much sugar encourages bacterial growth and can decrease immune function, setting the stage for infection. Eat healthful snacks that are low in sugar, especially if you are prone to bladder infections.

RQ 3 **Try herbal therapy.** Uva-ursi (*Arctostaphylos uva-ursi*) is an herb that helps to soothe, tone, and strengthen the membranes of the urinary system. Also, try buchu (*Barosma betulina*), an herb that has a diuretic effect and acts as an antiseptic to the urinary tract system. Both uva-ursi and buchu can be found at natural foods stores.

Eat yogurt. Studies suggest that lactobacilli, the active bacterial cultures in yogurt, help to prevent bladder infections. Make sure the label on your yogurt says that it contains live cultures.

Boost healing with essential nutrients. Take essential fatty acids—fish oil, flaxseed oil, evening primrose oil (*Oenothera biennis*), or borage oil (*Borago officinalis*)—and vitamin E to help boost tissue healing. Store them in a cool, dark place.

Increase antioxidants. Add daily supplements of vitamin C to protect against infection and aid in tissue healing. Vitamin C discourages the formation of free radicals, which cause damage to cells and impair the immune system. See "Dietary Reference Intakes" on page 164 for safe levels of vitamin C.

Add zinc. Zinc has tremendous antioxidant effects and is vital to your body for tissue repair. Many illnesses, including kidney disease and long-term infection, are associated with zinc deficiency. If you are taking certain medications, they may interfere with zinc absorption in the intestines and cause a zinc deficiency. While you should discuss taking any supplemental zinc with your doctor, to improve immune function, eat foods high in zinc including seafood, eggs, meats, whole grains, wheat germ, nuts, and seeds. Avoid coffee and tea, which are diuretics containing tannins that contract tissues and may hinder zinc absorption.

Soothe it. Try a sitz bath—a warm water bath that covers the lower abdomen, hips, and buttocks. For maximum effect, alternate between hot and cold baths, which helps improve pelvic circulation.

Avoid irritants. Avoid using tampons if you have a bladder infection or if you are prone to them since they can be irritating. Also avoid hygienic sprays, deodorizing or perfumed sanitary napkins, bubble baths, and perfumed soaps, as these can increase irritation.

When to Call the Doctor: If you notice bloody or cloudy urine, or if you have a frequent need to urinate yet can only eliminate a few drops, call your doctor for an evaluation because you may have a bacterial infection that requires antibiotics. If you experience lower back pain or have a high fever, contact your doctor immediately.

Blisters

What Is It? A blister is a raised area of skin, usually oval or circular in shape, which is filled with fluid. You can avoid a doctor's visit by treating a minor blister immediately. But if you have diabetes, check in with your doctor just to make sure that self-care is safe for your special condition.

What Causes It? Blisters form as a result of moisture, heat, and friction. The fluid inside is leaked from blood vessels in underlying skin layers after minor damage, such as a burn, skin disease, fungal infection, allergy, friction, or diseases such as chickenpox or shingles.

Signs and Symptoms: You will notice a raised portion of damaged skin that feels soft to the touch. To avoid infection, protect it from tearing by covering it loosely with a gauze bandage.

Prevention and Treatment:

RQ 1 **Stay well-hydrated.** Make sure you are drinking at least 8 glasses (64 ounces) of water or clear liquid each day to help protect skin, keep it hydrated, and aid in healing.

Eat your weedies. A well-balanced diet of fresh fruits and vegetables ensures your body of vitamins, minerals, and special nutrients called antioxidants and phytochemicals that are thought to help bolster immune function and keep you well.

Heal the wound. Use calendula ointment, found at most natural foods stores, to help with the healing of the blister before it bursts and after it has begun the healing process. *Calendula officinalis* is a flower that has been known for centuries as a natural healing and soothing substance when applied locally.

Take care. If you accidentally snag the blister, causing its liquid to secrete, be sure you keep it clean and loosely covered with a gauze bandage.

RQ 2 **Check your protein intake.** Protein is important in building and repairing body tissue and in fighting infection. Too little protein in the diet may lead to symptoms of fatigue, weakness, apathy, and poor immunity. An average adult needs 45 to 55 grams of protein each day, but you need more protein if you have a fever or infection. (But if you have renal failure and are not on dialysis, check with your doctor before increasing your dietary protein.) One ounce of lean meat, chicken, cheese, or fish provides 7 grams of protein; 1 cup of milk provides 8 grams of protein. Therefore, 5 to 6 ounces of meat per day and 2 cups of milk provide adequate protein for most adults. Vegetable proteins (legumes, beans, and tofu) can make a good substitute for animal protein when eaten as part of a properly balanced diet.

Up your essential fatty acids. Essential fatty acids (EFAs), such as those in flaxseed oil, cold pressed fish oil, cod-liver oil, evening primrose oil (*Oenothera biennis*), or black currant oil (*Ribes nigrum*), can help to boost your immune function. All of these can be found at most grocery and natural foods stores; store them in a cool, dark place.

RQ 3 **Use immune-boosting supplements.** Along with suggestions made for RQs 1 and 2, make sure you are getting adequate zinc, vitamin C, and B vitamins in your daily supplements (see "Dietary Reference Intakes" on page 164 for specific information).

Try an herbal cocktail. Two immune boosting herbs, echinacea (*Echinacea purpurea* or *E. angustifolia*) and garlic (*Allium sativum*), may help your blisters to heal quickly. Echinacea may fight bacterial and viral infections, while garlic is a known antimicrobial—important so the blister does not worsen.

RQ 4 **Use a healing oil.** Vitamin E oil can also speed healing when directly applied to superficial wounds. Use the oil-filled capsules or pure oil found at most grocery or natural foods stores.

Coat it with aloe gel. Break open an aloe (*Aloe barbadensis*) leaf and rub the sticky gel on the skin. Historically, aloe has been used for soothing burns, but it will promote the healing of blisters, too.

When to Call the Doctor: Blisters can be serious, particularly if they become infected. That's why a watchful eye is most important, along with use of the self-care tips in Risk Quotients 1 through 4. If the blister starts to expand, turns bright red, or there is a discharge (other than the liquid that would escape if you accidentally pricked the skin), see your doctor.

Boils

What Is It? Boils are inflamed, pus-filled nodules on the skin, usually on the shoulders, face, scalp, buttocks, or armpits. When they form into a cluster they're called carbuncles.

What Causes It? These nodules are generally caused by a staph infection.

Signs and Symptoms: Boils start in the hair follicles and are itchy red lumps that become painful. As they fill with pus, they become round and form a yellowish tip.

Prevention and Treatment:

RQ 1 **Be sanitary.** Keep the area clean by washing with a gentle cleanser and warm water several times a day. Avoid overwashing, as this may cause irritation. Use soft paper towels to wash the site of the boil, disposing of them immediately to avoid contamination. Dry the site with a separate paper towel. If you use washcloths, launder them separately and immediately to avoid infecting others in your household. Avoid touching or picking at the boil. Keep it covered with a gauze bandage to protect it from irritation.

Use preventive medicine. You can avoid spreading the staph infection by taking showers instead of baths, and use towels that no one else in the household will use.

Keep it warm. Use moist heat compresses every hour or two to help increase blood flow to the injured area, helping to speed healing.

Chill! Avoid stressful situations, as stress wreaks havoc with hormones and may lower your immune defenses. Learn how to work periods of time-out or relaxation into your daily routine to ease tension and give your body time to recover.

RQ 2 **Shun irritants.** Avoid perfumed soaps, strong deodorants, and scratchy clothing that may irritate the infected area. Do not reuse a razor to shave underarms if you've had an outbreak of boils.

This can make the infection spread rapidly to other areas of the body. If someone else used your razor, they, too, could experience boils.

Stay regular. Make sure you have regular bowel movements, at least one or two per day, so toxins and hormones are properly eliminated. A diet high in fiber and complex carbohydrates can help to eliminate toxins. You could also try acidophilus (*Lactobacillus acidophilus*) to help ensure proper gastrointestinal metabolism; it can be purchased in natural foods stores.

RQ 3

Invest in natural supplements. Consider taking zinc, vitamin C, and essential fatty acids (EFAs). (See "Dietary Reference Intakes" on page 164.) Zinc is known to fight infection, boost immune function, and help with hormone metabolism. Vitamin C helps ensure proper collagen formation and skin integrity. While not manufactured by the body, EFAs are essential to good health and are available in fish or flaxseed oils, which contain omega-3.

Eat foods high in vitamin E: Vitamin E is important to the body for the maintenance of cell membranes. Some studies reveal that foods high in vitamin E help to stimulate the function of T-cells, which are important fighters of the immune system. Food sources of vitamin E include almonds, lobster, corn oil, cod-liver oil, safflower oil, salmon, hazelnuts, and sunflower seeds.

RQ 4

Add vitamin A. Vitamin A is a super antioxidant that has been shown to boost healing in problem skin, as well as to protect the skin from the damaging effects of the sun's ultraviolet rays. Add foods high in vitamin A, such as carrots, sweet potatoes, apricots, cantaloupes, pumpkins, pink grapefruit, tomatoes, peaches, and collard greens, to your diet.

Try herbal therapies. Milk thistle (*Silybum marianum*) and dandelion (*Taraxacum officinale*) can help to detoxify the body. Goldenseal (*Hydrastis canadensis*), echinacea (*Echinacea purpurea* or *E. angustifolia*), and garlic (*Allium sativum*) can bolster immune function and help combat infection. These herbs are available at most grocery or natural foods stores.

Use natural healing. A poultice—a moist herbal preparation spread onto the affected area of the body and covered with a clean, dry cloth—can help. Apply a poultice made of 1 part apple cider vinegar and 10 parts filtered water to the affected area. Keep this away from eyes and other sensitive tissues, as it may burn.

When to Call the Doctor: Because a boil is a potentially dangerous staph infection, if it worsens after a day or two, call your doctor. If the boil is large, antibiotics may be necessary to help your body get rid of the infection. You may also need your doctor to open (lance) the boil to drain the pus. This is done using a sterile needle and will help to alleviate any pain.

Bronchitis

What Is It? Before you run to the doctor seeking antibiotics to treat bronchitis, think again. Acute bronchitis is an infection of the bronchial tubes frequently caused by viruses. When these tubes get infected, they swell, and mucus forms. Chronic bronchitis (also known as chronic obstructive pulmonary disease, or COPD) is a different type of bronchial infection that is usually associated with cigarette smoking and may worsen with air pollution, respiratory infections, or allergies.

What Causes It? This common respiratory condition can be an acute, or temporary, problem following a viral infection, or a chronic, long-term respiratory condition with a constant buildup of mucus and a productive cough.

The same viruses that cause colds often cause acute bronchitis, so antibiotics are not helpful, even when the mucus you cough up is yellow or thick. Sometimes, when your bronchial tubes are inflamed, you may develop a secondary infection, such as bacterial pneumonia or bacterial bronchitis, which needs a doctor's immediate attention and for which antibiotic treatment may be needed. You may get acute bronchitis from exposure to cigarette smoke or other pollutants such as household cleaners and smog. You may also develop bronchitis when the acids from your stomach back up into your esophagus, a condition known as gastroesophageal reflux disease (GERD).

Signs and Symptoms: With bronchitis, you may have a productive cough, thick or discolored mucus, fever, fatigue, wheezing, and shortness of breath. Other symptoms include soreness and a feeling of constriction in the chest. Sometimes chronic sinusitis—an ongoing infection in the lining of one or more of the cavities in the bones around your nose—may to some degree mimic bronchitis (called *sinobronchial syndrome*).

Prevention and Treatment:

RQ 1 **Use healing aromatherapy.** Breathe in aromatic steam. Fill the bathroom sink with steaming water and add 2 teaspoons chopped fresh ginger (*Zingiber officinale*). Drape a towel over your head and lean over the steam to get maximum benefit. Or add 1 teaspoon of the over-the-counter ointment Vicks VapoRub to the steaming water, then breathe in the steam for several minutes until you get relief. Another alternative is to add a few drops of eucalyptus (*Eucalyptus globulus*) essential oil or menthol to the water. Eucalyptus is known to open up bronchial tubes, ease congestion, and make breathing easier.

Liquefy thick mucus. Stay well-hydrated by drinking at least 8 glasses (64 ounces) of water each day. Water helps to keep your respiratory system hydrated, which aids in liquefying thick mucus that builds up to cause infection in your bronchial tubes. Other liquids can be added, but don't depend on coffee, tea, or alcoholic beverages, as these liquids dehydrate the body.

Take bromelain. Bromelain, the active component of pineapple, has been shown, in a 2001 study, to help ease inflammation and may prevent the progression of bronchitis in many patients. This supplement is available at most natural foods stores.

Avoid triggers. Avoid all airway irritants including pollen, airborne allergens, and dust from tissues. If possible, use a high-efficiency particulate air (HEPA) filter vacuum cleaner, which removes a far greater degree of minute particles than an ordinary vacuum. Wash your hair prior to bed to rid your head of pollen that will aggravate the condition while sleeping. Eliminate all down/feather pillows and comforters, which can also cause reactions. Do not allow pets into the bedroom during your illness until it is resolved. Do not keep your home so warm as to dry out mucous membranes, which can cause a decreased resistance to illness. Use a humidifier if the air in your home is dry, and make sure to clean your humidifier daily to prevent molds and fungi from building up. Dust at least once or twice a week, and damp-mop all hardwood floors. Avoid any of your known food allergens.

RQ 2

Make mullein tea. This herb has expectorant qualities that can quickly ease a dry bronchial cough. Mullein (*Verbascum thapsus*) contains the active plant constituents mucilage (which coats the respiratory tract, soothing mucous membranes and protecting against irritation), saponins (strong expectorants), and tannins (which improve resistance to infection). This herb brings up the sticky phlegm, soothes the scratchy throat, and has antibacterial action. It also calms the bronchial muscle spasm that causes the constant coughing. You can find mullein tea at natural foods stores. Since mullein is bitter in taste, you may want to add honey to sweeten.

Control inflammation. The key to resolving bronchitis is to control the inflammation, keep the airways sufficiently moist, and prevent the bronchial muscle spasms that cause coughing. Ginger (*Zingiber officinale*) has been used for medicinal purposes in China for thousands of years. It has antioxidant and anti-inflammatory effects, and it stimulates the production of interferon, which helps fight viral infections.

Use deep abdominal breathing. If you are prone to getting respiratory problems, it's important to practice deep breathing several times a day to ensure that the airway stays oxygenated. Here's what to do: Lie on your back in a quiet room with no distractions. Place your hands on your abdomen, then slowly and deliberately breathe in through your nostrils. If your hands are rising and your abdomen is expanding, then you are breathing correctly. If your hands do not rise yet you see your chest rising, you are breathing incorrectly.

Boost immune function: A 1999 study from Germany suggests that echinacea (*Echinacea purpurea* or *E. angustifolia*) may mildly stimulate the immune system and help to ward off colds and respiratory infections.

RQ 3 **Breathe clean air.** Get a HEPA filter or humidifier for your home. A HEPA filter, found at most department, discount, and hardware stores, is efficient in filtering out almost 100 percent of airborne allergens and particle irritants. Also use a mild peroxide solution (see page 250) to eliminate mold and mildew in showers, basements, windowsills, and dark rooms. Clean your humidifier daily to prevent the build up and spread of molds and fungi.

Get pungent protection. Onions and scallions, horseradish, radishes, and hot peppers may stimulate respiratory mucus production, which can help eliminate microbes from the body. Onions and scallions contain quercetin, a plant chemical that has been found to block allergic reactions by inhibiting the release of histamine and prostaglandins.

Make thyme tea. This immune-boosting herb (*Thymus vulgaris*) contains the phytochemical thymol and has been used in antiseptic mouthwashes and herbal cough remedies. It is also used in herbal teas, especially for treating mild symptoms associated with coughs, bronchitis, or colds.

Add immune-boosting herbs. Take goldenseal (*Hydrastis canadensis*) to soothe inflammation of the respiratory tract caused by allergy or infection. It's believed that goldenseal enhances mucous membrane function and increases immune function. Also take astragalus (*Astragalus membranaceus*) to stimulate white blood cell activity and increase the production of interferon, an antiviral agent. Thought to bolster resistance to disease, this herb is high in flavonoids, which are the anti-inflammatory active plant constituents.

Eat hot chicken soup. Hot chicken soup, sometimes known as grandma's penicillin, is a potent mucus stimulant, especially when it's loaded with pepper, garlic, hot curry powder, or other pungent spices that help to thin mucus in the mouth, throat, and lungs.

RQ 4

Spice it up. Chili peppers are a great source of capsaicin, an antioxidant that also acts as a natural decongestant and expectorant. Season your food with cayenne or hot sauce to open your sinuses and improve breathing.

Keep mucus thin. When mucus gets thick and stagnates, it causes bacteria to breed and increases the chance of infection. With bronchitis, keep mucus flowing by taking expectorants such as guaifenesin, which is found in over-the-counter cough products such as Robitussin.

Eat fish. Researchers believe that eating high-fat fish such as mackerel, cod, or salmon that are rich in omega-3 fatty acids tends to decrease inflammation. Besides omega-3s, salmon is filled with calcium, magnesium, some carotenoids (powerful antioxidants that are responsible for the color of red, orange, and yellow fruits and vegetables), complete proteins, and B vitamins. Vitamin B_6 supports immune function and has been shown in some preliminary tests to reduce breathing problems.

When to Call the Doctor: If your symptoms worsen, or if you have shortness of breath, wheezing, blood-streaked mucus, fever higher than 101° F, or vomiting, call your doctor, who may take a chest x-ray to make sure no pneumonia is present or blood tests to measure oxygen levels in your blood. Occasionally sputum may be obtained for culture to determine the cause of the bronchitis.

Burns

What Is It? A burn is damage on the skin that results in redness, blisters, and peeling. Burns can be very minor, but serious burns can lead to life-threatening infection if not carefully treated and monitored. More than 1 million people report burns each year in the United States.

What Causes It? The common causes of burns on the skin include heat, friction, sunlight, electricity, chemical irritants, or loss of moisture.

Signs and Symptoms: It's important to distinguish a minor burn from a more severe burn. Examine the extent of damage to the skin, using these three classifications to evaluate your burn and to determine the level of care necessary:

- First-degree (superficial): A minor burn in which the outer or top layer of skin (epidermis) is injured, such as when you have a moderate sunburn. Your skin is red, swollen, painful to touch, and may peel off in 1 or 2 days. A superficial burn usually heals within 1 week.

- Second-degree (superficial, partial thickness): A more serious burn in which both the top or outer layer of skin (epidermis) and second layer of skin (dermis) are burned through. Your skin is bright red with a blister covering the injury. You will have constant and severe pain and swelling. A second-degree burn usually takes 2 to 3 weeks to heal.
- Third-degree (full thickness): A severe burn damaging all skin layers, resulting in charred or white skin. Third-degree burns might not be painful because the nerves may be destroyed. They typically take more than 3 weeks to heal.

Severe second-degree, all third-degree, and all electrical burns require immediate medical treatment. You should seek medical advice if you are unable to classify your burn or if the burn covers a large area of skin.

Prevention and Treatment:

RQ 1 **Cool the burn.** Immediately cool the burn by placing it under cool water for 10 to 15 minutes (ice or ice water may further damage your skin). Or place cold cloths or compresses on top of the burn, which helps to reduce inflammation.

Stay hydrated. Drink plenty of water.

Hands off. The best protection you can give your burn is to leave any blisters intact. Move carefully to avoid popping the blister and keep the skin clean during this healing process. If you need to cover the burn, use a thin layer of wet gauze but do not allow the gauze to stick to the burn. Avoid using cotton balls on the burn because they have a tendency to stick to moist skin and may irritate the burn.

RQ 2 **Coat it with aloe.** For first- and second-degree burns, use aloe gel or a crushed aloe leaf (*Aloe barbadensis*) to help resolve pain and speed healing.

Elevate. It's important to keep the burned area elevated to help prevent swelling by reducing blood flow to the area, which encourages your body's natural healing.

Add immune-boosting therapy. Boost your immune-fighting cells with vitamin C, echinacea (*Echinacea purpurea* or *E. angustifolia*), and goldenseal (*Hydrastis canadensis*).

Prevent infection. After cleaning the burn, coat it with an over-the-counter antibacterial cream such as Neosporin to prevent infection. Cover with a loose gauze bandage and watch for signs of infection: increased redness, increased pain, pus, or swelling. If you notice these signs, call your doctor.

Check your immunization record. Burns can become infected, so make sure you are current on your tetanus shot, especially with more severe second- or third-degree burns.

When to Call the Doctor: Watch for signs of infection, such as increased pain, redness, fever, swelling, or oozing. Infection will cause poor healing and further damage. If infection develops, get medical help immediately. Severe second-degree, all third-degree, and electrical burns require immediate medical treatment.

Canker Sores

What Is It? Canker sores, also known as aphthous ulcers, are small, craterlike sores inside the mouth that usually last from 10 to 14 days. These tiny, oval, reddish swellings occur on the movable parts of your mouth—the tongue, soft palate, and inside your cheeks. While canker sores usually appear infrequently, some people are plagued with them up to 50 percent of the time.

What Causes It? The actual cause of canker sores is unknown. Some people have a genetic predisposition to getting these painful mouth ulcers, while others may feel canker sores after a mouth injury or scrape. Canker sores may have an immune system link and may be associated with periods of great stress, hormonal fluctuations, nutritional deficiencies, and food allergies. Some researchers hypothesize that certain foods—for example, citrus fruits, pineapples, tomatoes, and some nuts—may complicate the problem and add to your misery.

Canker sores differ from cold sores in that they occur in the soft tissues of your mouth and aren't contagious. Conversely, cold sores are viral and extremely contagious, and they rarely develop in those areas of your mouth.

Signs and Symptoms: While very tiny and hard to see, canker sores are painful and annoying. After about a day, the swellings rupture and are coated with a thin yellow or white membrane. The sores can be an eighth of an inch wide to more than 1 inch wide in serious cases. You may feel unresolved pain and burning for a few days, or have fatigue, swollen lymph nodes, and fever with more serious cases of mouth ulcers.

Prevention and Treatment:

RQ 1 **Watch what you eat!** If you are prone to getting canker sores, avoid foods that are abrasive (bagels, crackers), acidic (pineapples, tomatoes), or spicy (chili peppers), as they may irritate your mouth. Avoid foods rich in the amino acid arginine (nuts, seeds, and chocolate) until your mouth is healed, as arginine can aggravate the condition.

Gently brush your teeth. Be cautious when you brush your teeth, always using a soft toothbrush, to avoid tearing your gums or traumatizing your mouth. Change toothpaste if your gums are sensitive and the one you are using irritates your mouth.

Ice it. Apply ice to canker sores to ease the pain.

RQ 2 **Take an amino acid.** Consider supplementing with the amino acid lysine, which speeds healing. Food sources of lysine include cheese, eggs, fish, red meat, lima beans, potatoes, soy products, and yeast.

RQ 3 **Add pain-soothing herbal therapies.** Apply licorice (*Glycyrrhiza glabra*) extract to the affected area. Licorice is known to be high in flavonoids and antioxidants and can help to decrease inflammation. You may also apply lemon balm (*Melissa officinalis*) cream to the area. To speed healing, use coenzyme Q_{10} (CoQ_{10}) sublingually (under the tongue) or a sublingual vitamin B_{12}/folic acid tablet.

RQ 4 **Treat the inflammation.** Go to your favorite natural foods store and ask for a myrrh (*Commiphora myrrha*) product for that canker sore. Myrrh can be used as a mouthwash, or the dried herb can be mixed with water and applied to the sore. Germany's Commission E (a panel that authored one of the most comprehensive expert guides to therapeutic herbs ever produced) has endorsed powdered myrrh for treating inflammation in the mouth and throat because it contains tannins. Tannins are an antiseptic with antibacterial and antiviral properties and are helpful for mouth sores that may be caused by a virus, allergy, fungus, or bacterium.

When to Call the Doctor: If you experience an extremely painful, persistent, or large sore, or have difficulty eating or drinking, call your doctor for an evaluation. You may need a prescription medication such as an anesthetic solution or corticosteroid salve to help with pain and swelling.

Colds

What Is It? A cold is a *viral* infection of the upper respiratory tract—which is why it generally isn't useful to ask your doctor for antibiotics to treat the cold's misery. Lingering cold symptoms, however, may indicate a bacterial infection elsewhere in your body such as your ears, lungs, or sinuses. For this reason, colds are included in this rundown of common illnesses.

What Causes It? Although more than 200 viruses can cause colds, the culprit is usually the rhinovirus, Respiratory Syncytial Virus (RSV). Cold viruses enter your body through your nose or mouth and can be spread by touching someone who's sick or sharing common objects and then touching your nose or mouth. If you aren't cautious about hand washing and covering your nose and mouth when you sneeze and cough, you can spread your cold to others. While most colds last about a week, if your symptoms continue, you may have a bacterial infection.

Most children get their first colds before age 1. Colds spread rapidly in close quarters such as day care settings and school classrooms. Adults generally get colds less frequently than children.

Signs and Symptoms: You may feel an itchy or sore throat with sneezing, nasal congestion, watery eyes, and profuse mucus drainage. You may also have aches, headache, fatigue, and sometimes a low-grade fever (below 101° F). Through the course of the cold, the nasal mucus will become thicker and discolored.

Prevention and Treatment:

RQ 1 **Practice prevention.** Avoiding colds is possible by paying attention to your own health and the health of those around you. If you see someone who is obviously sick, keep your distance.

When a cold strikes you or your child, you can make a big difference in stopping the spread of colds by staying home and keeping your child at home. Don't share tubes of toothpaste, store toothbrushes separately to avoid spreading germs, and get a new toothbrush once the illness has passed. For most colds, treating these viral infections with antibiotics won't help. In the current medical system, however, many physicians will prescribe an antibiotic if it is not clear that the symptoms are the result of a viral infection or if the patient insists. Your doctor will probably have a good idea about what's going around, so let your doctor advise you about appropriate treatment before you start insisting on antibiotics.

Stay well-hydrated. Keep the heat turned down to 68° F or below, and if the air is dry or if you are experiencing dry skin, consider running a humidifier. Make sure to clean your humidifier daily to prevent molds and fungi from building up. Also, drink 8 glasses of water each day.

Think zinc. There are some exciting studies that suggest sucking on zinc lozenges at the start of a cold may lessen its severity. One study at Dartmouth College in Hanover, New Hampshire, reported that students who took zinc lozenges at the onset of a cold had only 5 days of symptoms, compared with 9 days for students who received placebos (no medication). These results may be because the zinc has an antiviral effect in the mouth and nose. Researchers from Wayne State University School of Medicine in Detroit have suggested that zinc fosters immunity. The body may be unable to fight infection without sufficient supplies of this nutrient. While these small studies are encouraging, the jury is still out on zinc's effectiveness. The best way to ingest zinc safely is through foods such as oysters, almonds, meat, milk, black-eyed peas, sunflower seeds, tofu, wheat germ, and crabmeat.

Add natural healers. Boost your intake of foods high in vitamin C when you've been exposed to a cold. Vitamin C (ascorbic acid) protects us against infection and aids in healing. A study in the *New England Journal of Medicine* found that psychological stress increased susceptibility to the common cold. While there is no direct research in evaluating vitamin C in preventing colds, studies have shown that the vitamin may lessen both the symptoms and the duration of a cold. Foods high in vitamin C include broccoli, cantaloupes, cauliflower, papayas, peppers (red, green, or yellow), kale, kiwifruit, sweet potatoes, tomatoes, oranges, and strawberries.

RQ 2 **Increase rest and healing sleep.** Plan rest times throughout the day to give your body a chance to gain strength. Also getting enough deep healing sleep will allow your body tissues to rejuvenate and boost immune function.

Keep your hands washed. When your immune system is depleted during an illness, it's easy to get another germ. You can avoid self-inoculation (giving yourself bad germs) by keeping your hands washed regularly and refraining from touching your face. As discussed in chapter 2, only about half of people wash their hands after using public bathrooms, so avoid faucets and doorknobs in these areas if possible, or touch them using paper towels.

RQ 3 **Take the thyme.** Add common thyme (*Thymus vulgaris*) to your daily supplement regimen. Thyme contains thymol, which is a phytochemical. This immune-boosting herb has been used in antiseptic mouthwashes and herbal cough remedies. It is also used in herbal teas, especially for treating mild symptoms associated with colds, flu, or coughs.

Try a nighttime nasal strip to ease symptoms. If nasal swelling and congestion keep you from sleeping soundly at night, nasal strips may help to alleviate this problem. These strips of tape are placed over the bridge of the nose, then a plastic strip springs back, helping to gently open your nasal passages and reduce airflow resistance. Another method to encourage nighttime breathing is to use ¼-inch wide surgical tape. Gently apply one end of the tape to the tip of your nose, lift, and fasten the other end of the tape to the top of your nose.

RQ 4 **Use an over-the-counter nasal spray.** If you want immediate relief for a swollen, congested nasal passage, decongestant nasal sprays such as oxymetazoline (Afrin) and phenylephrine (Neo-Synephrine) may be helpful. Decongestant nasal sprays are safe to use to halt the progression of sinus infections following colds, but it's important to stop the spray after 3 to 5 days to avoid the development of rebound congestion. If you have high blood pressure or narrow angle glaucoma, then you should seek medical advice before taking any decongestants.

Opt for saline nasal sprays. Unlike the medicated nasal sprays, the saline nasal sprays can be used as often as necessary. They do not carry the same risk of rebound nasal congestion.

Drink up. Increase your fluid intake.

Spice it up. Chili peppers are a great source of capsaicin, an antioxidant that also acts as a natural decongestant and expectorant. You can try chili peppers to season your foods or use a few drops of hot sauce in a food or beverage to open your congested nasal passages and improve breathing.

Keep mucus thin. When mucus gets thick and stagnates, it causes bacteria to breed and increases the chance of infection. Keep mucus flowing by taking expectorants such as guaifenesin, which is found in over-the-counter cough products such as Robitussin. Also avoid any known food allergens.

When to Call the Doctor: If your symptoms have substantially worsened after the 5th day, if symptoms persist for more than 10 days, or if you have a fever of 101° F or higher, call your doctor to see whether you might have a secondary infection such as a sinus or ear infection, strep throat, bronchitis, or pneumonia. If you have fever, chills, sweating, and a productive cough, you could have pneumonia, which warrants immediate medical treatment. While antibiotics are not useful against cold viruses, they may be necessary for treating secondary infections.

Conjunctivitis

What Is It? Although conjunctivitis occurs most often in children, this highly contagious condition is of concern to adults as well. It happens when the conjunctiva, a transparent membrane that lines the inside of the eyelid and covers the whites of the eye, becomes inflamed.

What Causes It? Conjunctivitis can be caused by allergies, dry eyes, irritation, a virus, or a bacterial infection known as *pinkeye*, which is common in childcare centers and crowded classrooms. Both viral and bacterial conjunctivitis are contagious.

Signs and Symptoms: Symptoms include redness, tearing, a "gritty" feeling when blinking, itching, burning, and swelling of the eye and eyelid. With bacterial conjunctivitis, there is usually a thick, yellow-green, mucuslike discharge that glues the eyelid together. Viral conjunctivitis usually affects both eyes, while bacterial pinkeye may affect only one eye. Allergic conjunctivitis leaves the eyes red, itchy, and watery, but there is no thick, yellow-green discharge.

Prevention and Treatment:

RQ 1 **Keep the eye clean.** Use a clean moist tissue to dab the discharge away from the irritated eye. Use a clean tissue to dab the other eye, if needed. Discard the tissue immediately, and wash your hands to avoid spreading the infection.

Separate yourself. Do not use the same bar of soap, hand towels, or bath towels as others in your household. If you have bacterial conjunctivitis, you may be contagious for 2 days after treatment with antibiotics begins. Make sure to wash your hands frequently and use the antibiotics prescribed as directed. If your doctor believes that an allergy is causing the conjunctivitis, ask about using over-the-counter antihistamine eye drops such as Visine-A to ease the itching and inflammation. If your doctor confirms that a virus is causing the problem, ask about saline eye drops such as Visine or Tears Naturale to ease the discomfort. Never touch the tip of the dropper to the eye, as germs can spread to the product and infect others.

RQ 2 **Use moist heat compresses.** Warm, moist compresses can help to alleviate the inflammation that causes the pain and itching. Apply a compress to the eye every 3 or 4 hours to ease burning, and wipe away crusts. If applying to both eyes, use a clean cloth for the second eye. Never reuse the same compress; place immediately into the laundry and wash your hands to avoid spreading the infection.

RQ 3 RQ 4 Work with your doctor.

When to Call the Doctor: If you suspect conjunctivitis, contact your doctor to determine the cause because all that's red in the eye is not conjunctivitis—it could be iritis or other disorders in the eye that could lead to blindness if left untreated. Contact your doctor if you have blurred vision, heavy eye tearing, thick mucus in the eye, or fever. Only your doctor can determine which type of conjunctivitis you have, and the treatment differs depending on whether it's viral or bacterial. Rare types of conjunctivitis can lead to blindness if left untreated.

Cough

What Is It? Cough is one of the most prevalent symptoms of nose and lung airway diseases, and it's extremely common. In fact, this sudden forceful release of air from the throat is the body's defense mechanism, helping to rid the body of any foreign material, irritation, or obstruction. A cough can last for a week, or it may extend for weeks or months, depending on the cause.

What Causes It? Cough stems from many different causes, like postnasal drip, chronic allergic rhinitis, sinusitis, or gastroesophageal reflux (heartburn). Asthma is a relatively common, serious cause of cough. Infections, such as bronchitis and pneumonia, can also cause cough. These infections may be bacterial, viral, or fungal. Smoking is yet another serious cause of cough, as it destroys the lining of the breathing tubes so mucus cannot be expelled properly.

Signs and Symptoms: You may have a dry, nagging, unproductive cough or a productive cough that brings up phlegm or mucus. Sometimes wheezing accompanies cough, signaling an obstruction in the lungs or bronchial tubes. A cough that just won't go away could be a symptom of another serious respiratory disease warranting medical attention.

Prevention and Treatment:

RQ 1 **Avoid smoking and smoke-filled environments.** Smoke contains irritants that can trigger cough and exacerbate existing conditions such as asthma. This includes wood-burning stoves, so limit your exposure to them when you have a cough.

Keep mucus thin. Drink plenty of water daily.

Run the humidifier. If the air is dry, a warm-mist humidifier or vaporizer can moisten the air and help ease coughing and any congestion. Be sure to keep the humidifier clean, however, to prevent the growth of bacteria, molds, and fungi.

Add an expectorant. An expectorant is a mucus mobilizer, helping to thin thick mucus, making it easier to cough it up. An effective expectorant is guaifenesin, which is found in Robitussin and other over-the-counter cough syrups. Drinking water and eating spicy foods also helps to thin mucus so it can be expelled.

RQ 2 **Try herbal remedies.** Take mullein (*Verbascum thapsus*), ginger (*Zingiber officinale*), and licorice (*Glycyrrhiza glabra*) to help thin mucus. These three healing herbs are known to be natural expectorants, helping to thin thick secretions so the body can expel them. Licorice cough drops are available over-the-counter. The ingredients in licorice cough drops aid in soothing scratchy throats and alleviating dry coughs.

RQ 3 **Try lozenges.** Sucking on soothing lozenges will help to moisten and coat the throat and reduce the cough. Sucking on zinc lozenges (especially zinc-gluconate with glycine) at the start of a cold may lessen its severity and reduce the subsequent cough (see "Colds," page 111).

Consider saline nasal drops. These salt water drops can be purchased over-the-counter and are effective, safe, and nonirritating. Put several drops into one nostril, then gently blow your nose. Repeat the process in the opposite nostril until both are running clear.

RQ 4 **Get pungent protection.** Onions and scallions, horseradish, radishes, and hot peppers may stimulate respiratory mucus production, which can help eliminate microbes from the body. Onions and scallions contain quercetin, a plant chemical that has been found to block allergic reactions by inhibiting the release of histamine and prostaglandins.

When to Call the Doctor: While short-lasting coughs (1 week) are okay to self-treat, if you have a cough that persists for more than 2 weeks, see your doctor. You may have a respiratory infection, allergy, asthma, or "walking" pneumonia. If you are coughing up blood, have shortness of breath, or have experienced a fever, sudden weight loss, and fatigue, see your doctor for immediate treatment.

Cuts and Scratches

What Is It? Cut, scratches, and other wounds are lacerations (openings or breaks in the skin) caused by physical injury.

What Causes It? There can be many causes of breaks in the skin from a cut, puncture, or tear to a scrape or splinter. In elderly adults, the skin sometimes tears for the smallest reason because it is so thin. Bacteria can cause a wound to become infected.

Signs and Symptoms: You will see the skin torn or open, along with blood and injured tissue. Most of the time, cuts and scratches are painful. With some wounds, you may not have a lot of pain, even though the wound is more serious.

Prevention and Treatment:

RQ 1 **Take precautions.** It's important to keep all wounds—large or small—clean and dry and to allow small wounds to bleed for a minute to get rid of infectious agents. Keep up-to-date with tetanus shots.

Hands off. To cover the wound after cleaning, use a thin layer of antibacterial cream such as Neosporin or an antiseptic spray like Bactine and loosely cover with gauze. Try not to let the gauze stick to the open wound or it may cause irritation.

RQ 2 **Coat it with aloe.** Aloe gel or the sticky residue from a crushed aloe (*Aloe barbadensis*) leaf may help to resolve pain and speed healing.

Stay hydrated. Drink plenty of water to keep your skin hydrated and protected.

Elevate the wound. Keep the injured area elevated to help prevent swelling by reducing blood flow to the area and supporting your body's natural healing.

RQ 3 **Add immune-boosting therapy.** Boost your immune-fighting cells with echinacea (*Echinacea purpurea* or *E. angustifolia*) and goldenseal (*Hydrastis canadensis*).

RQ 4 **Invest in natural supplements.** Take zinc, vitamin C, and essential fatty acids (EFAs). (See "Dietary Reference Intakes" on page 164.) Zinc helps to fight infection. Vitamin C helps to ensure proper collagen formation and skin integrity. EFAs are not manufactured by the body but are essential to good health and are available in fish and flaxseed oils, which contain omega-3.

When to Call the Doctor: If a wound is a puncture or is deep or bleeding profusely, seek immediate medical help. If the wound begins to secrete a liquid or oozes after a few days of self-care, continues to bleed, has an odor, or forms a damp yellow or green scab, call your doctor. You may have an infection that needs medical treatment.

Diarrhea

What Is It? Diarrhea is an unpleasant digestive disorder that affects about 10 percent of people once a year. The loose-stool consistency usually lasts a few days at most. Diarrhea often means more frequent trips to the bathroom and may mean your stool is greater in volume.

What Causes It? The most common causes of loose, watery stools and abdominal cramps are infections from bacteria, viruses, or parasites. Certain bacteria can make a toxin that triggers intestinal cells to secrete rather than to absorb salt and water. This overwhelms the capacity of your lower small bowel or your colon—or both—to absorb fluid. The result is diarrhea.

You can spread diarrhea to others when you touch the stool of an infected person or something that is contaminated with the stool of an infected person. Then if you touch your mouth with the contaminated hand, you are a prime candidate for diarrhea. Diarrhea is also transmitted through food or water contaminated with bacteria or parasites. In some cases, diarrhea is a symptom of another digestive disorder, such as irritable bowel syndrome, Crohn's disease, ulcerative colitis, celiac disease, or lactose intolerance.

Signs and Symptoms: You may have loose or watery stools, abdominal cramps and pain, nausea, and vomiting. If you have a bacterial or parasitic infection, you may have blood in the stools, and you may get a fever.

Prevention and Treatment:

RQ 1 **Focus on prevention.** You can help prevent the spread of diarrhea by washing your hands and encouraging your family members to do the same all the time, and especially when using public restrooms.

Watch what (and how) you eat. You can help prevent the spread of food-borne disease by carefully checking the expiration dates on foods, properly preparing and storing foods, and keeping hot foods hot and cold foods cold. Choose foods that are likely to be cooked well when you eat at restaurants.

Replenish lost fluid. After allowing the diarrhea to run its course for 8 to 12 hours, start replenishing lost fluid. Drink at least 8 glasses of clear liquids (water, broth, gelatin, juices, electrolyte replacement drinks such as CeraLyte or Oralyte, or weak decaffeinated tea) to prevent dehydration and replace much-needed electrolytes in the body. Do not drink alcohol or caffeine.

Sip decaffeinated tea. Sometimes it seems as if diarrhea will never run its course. And while it seems reasonable to cut your intake of fluids, drinking hot tea will help to calm your bowels and keep you from getting dehydrated during the illness. Tannins found in tea act as an astringent, reducing intestinal inflammation.

RQ 2 **Use safe food preparation.** Serve food immediately or keep it cold after it's been cooked or reheated. When you leave food out at room temperature, it encourages growth of bacteria.

Try the B.R.A.T. diet. If you get diarrhea, take an antidiarrheal medication to prevent excessive fluid loss (if recommended by your doctor). Once your diarrhea has subsided, ease back into eating your normal varied diet. For the first day after you have diarrhea, try a diet of bananas, rice, applesauce, and dry toast (B.R.A.T.). This bland diet is easily digested and will not irritate your sensitive gastrointestinal system. Stay away from milk or dairy products for a day or two, as it may add to your stomach discomfort.

Avoid unsafe foods. Avoid salad bars or buffet foods where people can touch utensils or foods. Don't eat raw or undercooked meats or dairy products that have not been refrigerated (such as at a picnic).

Add alternative therapies. Many people find good results by taking acidophilus (*Lactobacillus acidophilus*) or *Bifidobacterium bifidum* to replenish the body with good bacteria. Lactic acid bacteria are often called *probiotics* and serve to maintain the health of the intestinal tract by producing acids and other compounds that inhibit the growth of disease-causing bacteria.

RQ 3 **Slow down the bowels.** To help calm the irritated gastrointestinal system and slow down the bowels, some people find that taking Pepto-Bismol, Imodium A-D, or supplementing with betonite clay is helpful. Ask your doctor whether these might be right for you.

Add natural therapy. Take goldenseal (*Hydrastis canadensis*) to help kill harmful bacteria that may be causing the diarrhea.

RQ 4 **Increase fiber.** Work on keeping your bowels more regular. After the diarrhea episode is resolved, increase fiber intake in the diet or by stirring *psyllium husks* or another fiber product like Metamucil into water and drinking. Psyllium is a grain grown in India that is often used as a fiber supplement. But if you have a history of diverticulitis, avoid small seeds and nuts in your diet.

Boost bulk. Pectin, a soluble fiber found in apple peel, adds bulk to the stool, which can help to end diarrhea. Add cool applesauce to your diet. It not only tastes good when you are under the weather, but it helps to calm your intestines.

When to Call the Doctor: If diarrhea persists for more than a few days, it can cause you to become dehydrated, losing significant water and salts. Call your doctor if you cannot keep liquids down, have a fever higher than 101° F, are dizzy, fatigued, disoriented, or if you have severe, persistent abdominal or rectal pain, or bloody stools. Also, chronic or recurrent diarrhea may signal a more serious underlying medical problem such as chronic infection, inflammatory bowel disease, or poor absorption of nutrients.

Diverticulitis

What Is It? Nearly half of all Americans over age 60 have small, bulging pouches (diverticula) in their digestive tracts—a condition known as diverticulosis. Although diverticula can form anywhere, including your throat, stomach, and small intestine, most occur on the left side of your large intestine (colon). Because these pouches seldom cause any problems, you may never know you have them.

Sometimes, though, one or more pouches may become inflamed or infected, causing severe pain, fever, and nausea. When diverticula become infected, the condition is called diverticulitis. Mild cases of diverticulitis can be treated with changes in your diet, rest, and antibiotics. But more serious cases may require surgery to remove the diseased portion of your colon. Occasionally, you may develop complications that require emergency surgery.

What Causes It? Diverticula develop when naturally weak places in your colon wall give way under pressure. As a result, small pouches about the size and shape of a kernel of corn protrude through your colon wall. Pouches are most common in the descending colon and then the sigmoid colon, which ends just above your rectum. They often occur when you strain during a bowel movement.

If a small bit of stool becomes lodged in one of the pouches, it can cause infection. A small tear (perforation) can also develop in a pouch, leading to peritonitis (an infection of the lining of the outer bowel and wall of the abdomen) or pockets of pus (abscesses).

Signs and Symptoms: Diverticulitis can feel like appendicitis, except you'll have pain in the lower *left* side of your abdomen, instead of the lower right. The pain is usually severe and comes on suddenly, but sometimes you may have mild pain that becomes worse over several days. You may also have abdominal tenderness, fever, nausea, and either constipation or diarrhea.

Prevention and Treatment:

RQ 1 **Try a liquid diet.** Eat plenty of soups, broths, and other liquids during an attack. Avoid any foods containing small bits that could become trapped in the diverticula, such as seeds and nuts. If you are taking a diuretic, then talk to your doctor before trying this diet.

RQ 2 **Respond to bowel urges.** When you need to use the bathroom, do not delay. Delaying a bowel movement leads to harder stools that require more force to pass and increased pressure within your colon.

RQ 3 **Add more fiber.** Studies show that diverticulitis is rare in countries where people eat a high-fiber diet. That's because fiber holds water and helps keep your stool soft. In the United States, the average diet is high in refined carbohydrates and relatively low in fiber, so you might benefit from adding more fiber to your diet. Soluble fiber is abundant in fruits, oats, barley, and legumes, while insoluble fiber is found primarily in wheat bran, cereals, and vegetables.

Boost fluids. Because fiber works by absorbing water within your colon, if you don't drink enough liquid to replace what's absorbed, fiber can be constipating. Try to drink at least 8 glasses (64 ounces) of water or other beverages that don't contain caffeine or alcohol every day.

RQ 4 **Exercise regularly.** Exercise promotes normal bowel function and reduces pressure inside your colon. Try to exercise for at least 30 minutes on most days.

When to Call the Doctor: Diverticulitis can range from minor inflammation to a massive infection. Because it can be serious, see your doctor right away if you suspect you're having an attack. Unless your doctor tells you otherwise, don't eat anything (drinking is okay) and don't take a laxative. In rare cases, an infected or inflamed pouch in your intestine may rupture, spilling intestinal waste into your abdomen. This can lead to peritonitis, an inflammation of the lining of your abdominal cavity. Peritonitis is a medical emergency that requires immediate care.

Ear Infection

What Is It? Ear infection or otitis media, meaning inflammation of the middle ear, can occur in one or both ears. While not as common in adults as in children, it is often the result of inflamed and congested sinuses or a viral cold infection.

What Causes It? Fluid or pus build up in the middle ear, resulting in earache, swelling, and redness. Sometimes the eardrum ruptures, and the pus drains out of the ear. But more commonly, the pus and mucus remain in the middle ear due to the swollen and inflamed eustachian tube, a condition called middle ear effusion or serious otitis media. After the acute infection has passed, the effusion remains and becomes chronic, lasting for weeks, months, or even years. This condition makes you subject to frequent recurrences of the acute infection and may cause difficulty in hearing.

Any nasal congestion can cause an ear infection, especially when accompanied by a build-up of fluid, swollen mucous membranes, obstructions such as nasal polyps (grape-like growths inside the nasal cavity), or when you blow your nose too hard, closing the eustachian tube. A growth in the back of the nose can also press on the eustachian tube, blocking the normal flow of fluid, and allergies can cause inflammation that leads to infection.

Signs and Symptoms: With an ear infection, you will feel either a dull, throbbing pain or sharp, intense pains in the afflicted ear. You may have itching in the ear, and the outer lobe of the ear may be warm and red. Along with these symptoms, you could notice a decline in hearing capacity, as well as a buzzing sound or soft, high-pitched "ear noise" caused by pressure in the ear. With an infection, you may also have a fever, swollen glands, sore throat, sinus congestion, aches, and fatigue.

Prevention and Treatment:

RQ 1 **Stay hydrated.** Along with drinking at least 8 glasses of water (64 ounces), sip on hot black decaffeinated tea to help thin mucus and soothe inflammation.

Numb the pain. Use an analgesic to numb the pain of a beginning ear infection (the most painful part). You can use aspirin, acetaminophen (Tylenol), or a nonsteroidal anti-inflammatory drug (NSAID) like ibuprofen (Advil). The benefit of NSAIDs is that they decrease inflammation, the hidden cause of the ear pain, and give longer lasting relief than acetaminophen (6 hours compared to 4). If you cannot take these pain relievers, check with your doctor about another option to reduce pain.

RQ 2 **Avoid smoke.** Not only is cigarette smoke—both firsthand and secondhand—a trigger for mucus production and subsequent ear pain, but other sources such as wood stoves, fireplaces, and barbecue grills may cause problems.

RQ 3 RQ 4 **Use a mucus mobilizer.** Guaifenesin, the main ingredient in over-the-counter cough remedies such as Robitussin, works to keep mucus thin so it can flow freely in your nasal passages and eustachian tubes. This may help to alleviate discomfort and inflammation.

When to Call the Doctor: If your ear infection continues for 2 to 3 days with no relief, or if you have a fever higher than 101° F, swollen neck glands, sore throat, discharge from the ear, or dizziness, call your doctor. Sometimes, ear infections can cause disorientation and an inability to walk or stand, conditions for which medical treatment is necessary.

Fever

What Is It? Though a fever—an elevation in body temperature—is technically a symptom, it's in this list because it frequently accompanies a variety of infections, often sending us to the doctor to request antibiotics. Fever occurs when our body temperature rises to fight off infection. Normal body temperature is 98.6° F. When your temperature reaches 100° F or higher, you have a fever.

What Causes It? There are many reasons your body temperature might rise, including wearing warm clothes on a hot day or exercising vigorously. But the main cause of a fever is a bacterial or viral infection, including colds, flu, strep throat, gastrointestinal problems, respiratory infections, urinary tract infections, and even cancer.

A fever of up to 101° F in adults is tolerable for a couple of days. In fact, a fever is how your body tries to rid itself of microbes that do not survive well at these higher temperatures.

Signs and Symptoms: With a fever, you can feel extremely chilled, fatigued, and maybe even achy all over. Your eyes can burn or sting, and your mouth will feel dry or parched. You may have goose bumps, even though your skin is quite warm to the touch. A fever is called low-grade if it is 101° F or lower and high-grade if it is above 102° F.

Prevention and Treatment:

RQ 1 **Get more rest.** Getting plenty of rest and healing sleep is important to boost immune function and give the body time to heal. It is during the deeper stages of sleep that the healing process works best.

RQ 2 **Bathe in a tub of tepid water.** This will help to reduce your body temperature. Do not use cold water; it has no added benefit, may increase your chills, and can stress your body. Don't use ice cubes or rubbing alcohol to cool the body's temperature.

RQ 3 **Take an analgesic.** Acetaminophen (Tylenol) and ibuprofen (Advil) are known to reduce fever and alleviate body aches.

Increase fluids. With a fever, you can easily become dehydrated unless you are increasing fluids. Stick with water, clear broth, and electrolyte replacement drinks such as CeraLyte or Oralyte until the fever breaks.

RQ 4 Work with your doctor.

When to Call the Doctor: While a fever usually resolves with no medical treatment, call your doctor if you have a high-grade fever. If you have a stiff neck, severe headache, confusion or disorientation, sluggishness, or a purplish rash, or if there is another symptom associated with the fever (sore throat, earache, headache, difficulty urinating, gastrointestinal symptoms), call your doctor.

Flu

What Is It? The flu is a viral infection that mimics a cold except that it starts forcefully with symptoms of fatigue, fever, and respiratory congestion. While a cold is usually resolved within 1 week, it usually takes longer to get over the flu. This causes many people to request antibiotics from their doctor, hoping such treatments will offer quick relief. Although flus are viral, they can result in a secondary bacterial infection, such as pneumonia, that requires prescription medications.

What Causes It? The flu is actually quite different from a cold. While more than 100 different virus types can cause a cold, only influenza virus types A, B, and C cause the flu. Type A is constantly changing and is generally responsible for large flu epidemics, while types B and C are more stable and usually cause milder symptoms. The CDC develops a vaccine based on the type A strain that they believe will be most prevalent in the coming flu season, and this is what you receive if you get an annual flu shot; talk to your doctor.

Signs and Symptoms: The symptoms of the flu are similar to a cold, except you will feel them sooner and in greater intensity. You may feel extremely weak and fatigued, experience muscle aches, and go through periods of chills and sweats as the fever comes and goes. You will have a runny nose, headache, eye pain, and sore throat.

Prevention and Treatment:

RQ 1 **Stay in bed.** The first few days of the flu will hit you hard, and bed rest will let your body recover from the impact of symptoms.

Stay hydrated. Force fluids during the flu, including water, clear liquids, juices, broth soups, and electrolyte replacement drinks such as CeraLyte or Oralyte. Liquids help to thin mucus and replenish the body's fluids lost by fever. While you may not feel hungry or thirsty, liquids will keep you from getting dehydrated, which could worsen your body's condition. Do not drink alcohol or caffeine, as they act as diuretics and can upset the delicate balance of electrolytes in your body. You also need to get enough calories, so make sure you eat and drink enough to keep your strength.

Numb the pain. You can use aspirin, acetaminophen (Tylenol), or a nonsteroidal anti-inflammatory drug (NSAID) like ibuprofen (Advil). If you cannot take these pain relievers, check with your doctor about another option to reduce pain.

RQ 2 **Try herbal remedies.** While there is no instant cure for the flu, a few herbs may help to take the misery out of your symptoms. Elderberry (*Sambucus nigra*) is an ingredient in patent medicines in Israel, where one study showed that it decreases the duration of flu symptoms and prevents the flu virus from invading respiratory tract cells. Echinacea (*Echinacea purpurea* or *E. angustifolia*) is commonly used in Germany to ease symptoms and shorten duration of the flu. You may find even more relief with echinacea mixed with goldenseal (*Hydrastis canadensis*), which has a powerful antiviral action. Or, make ginger (*Zingiber officinale*) tea using 1 teaspoon fresh grated ginger root in 1 cup boiling water. Steep for 10 minutes, then strain.

Avoid smoke. Stop smoking and avoid secondhand smoke, including smoke from wood-burning stoves, as smoke can worsen your cold and respiratory symptoms.

Use saline nasal sprays. Saline nose sprays can help to ease the stuffiness, letting the clogged nasal passages open up again. When mucus stagnates in the nose and sinus cavity, it acts as a breeding ground for bacteria to grow, resulting in infection. Keep your passages clean and flowing to avoid this from happening.

RQ 3 **Use a mucus mobilizer.** Guaifenesin, the main ingredient in over-the-counter cough remedies such as Robitussin, works to keep mucus thin so it can flow freely in your nasal passages. This may help to alleviate discomfort and inflammation.

RQ 4 **Try papaya enzyme (papain) tablets.** These tablets, found at natural foods stores, are known to ease inflammation, resulting in thinner mucus. They are easily absorbed into the body if dissolved in your mouth between your cheek and gums.

Use a decongestant. Decongestants shrink the nasal passages and reduce congestion. Common ingredients of over-the-counter decongestants include phenylephrine and pseudoephedrine. (Do not take any medication containing phenylpropanolamine, as this has been found to cause stroke in some people, and consequently, this product has been removed from the market in the United States.)

Get the shot. Perhaps the best advice for those with RQ 4 is to get an annual flu shot. If you have chronic heart or lung disease, diabetes, kidney disease, immune system problems, or are over age 50, a flu shot can especially help you prevent problems in the first place. If you're pregnant with high-risk conditions, you might also want to consider a flu shot, but talk to your doctor first (especially if you are allergic to eggs).

When to Call the Doctor: If your flu symptoms worsen with fever of higher than 101° F, you cough up blood-stained mucus, or you experience difficulty breathing, wheezing, severe head pain, ear pain or drainage, difficulty swallowing, nausea and uncontrolled vomiting, or other unusual symptoms, call your doctor. The flu often goes into a secondary infection, such as pneumonia, which needs medical treatment. Also, if you have chronic obstructive pulmonary disease (COPD) or any form of lung disease, see your doctor at the first signs of flu to avoid complications. There are some prescription medications that may help to reduce symptoms if taken in the earliest stages of the flu.

Food Poisoning

What Is It? Food poisoning is increasingly becoming a 21st-century problem. Our busy lifestyles cause us to eat out more and seek convenient ready-to-eat prepared or fast foods. As I discuss in chapter 6, food poisoning may cause a brief stomachache for some of us, but others at higher risk can suffer more serious illness or even death.

What Causes It? Food-borne illness can result from viruses, parasites, fungi, and chemicals, but bacteria-related food poisoning, such as that caused by *Campylobacter* or *Salmonella*, is the most common. There are four factors that can rapidly increase the proliferation of bacteria to increase the chance of food poisoning.

1. Time: The longer food-poisoning pathogens stay alive, the greater their numbers. In some cases, over a period of 7 hours, more than two million bacteria can grow in food samples.

2. Temperature: Food-borne bacteria thrive when the temperature is in the "danger zone" between 40° and 140° F. As I explain in chapter 6, hot foods must be kept hot and cold foods must stay cold to keep these dangerous pathogens from breeding.

3. Nutrients: Certain foods are the perfect source for bacteria, providing them with the necessary nutrients to survive. Some of the most common bacterial breeding grounds include dairy foods, shellfish, eggs, meat, and poultry. Vegetables and fruits can also harbor food-borne pathogens if they come in contact with these bacteria during growth or processing.

4. Water: Food-borne bacteria must have moisture or water to survive. That's why it's important to keep food preparation surfaces dry to reduce the bacteria count.

Signs and Symptoms: Most of the symptoms of food poisoning are gastrointestinal, including nausea, vomiting, stomach pain, and cramping. You may also have fever, headache, and swollen lymph glands, depending on the type of bacteria. Those at high risk, including those with Risk Quotients of 4 or 5, pregnant women, infants, undernourished and immune-compromised people, and older adults, are at increased risk of experiencing serious symptoms resulting from food poisoning.

Prevention and Treatment: While food can easily become contaminated during processing, storage, and preparation, there are steps you can take to avoid becoming a victim.

- Wash your hands thoroughly both before and after preparing foods.

Signs of Dehydration

- Sunken eyes
- Light-headedness and increased thirst
- Dry or sticky mucous membranes in the mouth
- Lack of normal elasticity in the skin
- Decreased urine output
- Decreased tears

• Use separate cutting boards—one for raw animal products, and one for other foods such as vegetables, fruits, and breads—and sterilize the one for raw meats after use with the techniques in chapter 5.

• Cook and store foods at the appropriate temperatures (see chapter 6).

• Purchase the freshest foods possible, and dispose of foods that are past their expiration dates on the cartons. A good rule of thumb for food safety is "When in doubt, throw it out!"

RQ 1 **Do not induce vomiting.** Vomiting will not eliminate the food-borne bacteria. If you are healthy, the illness should run its course in a few days.

Stay hydrated. Drink plenty of liquids such as water, clear broths, electrolyte replacement drinks like CeraLyte or Oralyte, or diluted juices to avoid dehydration.

RQ 2 **Take an antidiarrheal medication.** To prevent excessive fluid loss, talk to your doctor about taking a medication like Imodium A-D or another antidiarrheal medication. Once your diarrhea has subsided, ease back into eating your normal diet.

Sip decaffeinated tea. Drinking warm tea will help to calm your bowels and keep you from getting dehydrated during the food-borne illness. Tannins found in tea act as an astringent, reducing intestinal inflammation.

Use the B.R.A.T. diet. For the first day after you have diarrhea, try a diet of bananas, rice, applesauce, and dry toast. This bland diet is easily digested and in unlikely to irritate your sensitive gastrointestinal system.

RQ 3 **Try an herbal remedy.** Ask your doctor about taking goldenseal (*Hydrastis canadensis*) or Oregon grape (*Mahonia aquifolium*) to help kill both food-borne bacteria and bacteria in the intestinal tract that may be sensitive to these herbs.

RQ 4 **Replace the good bacteria.** You may want to take acidophilus (*Lactobacillus acidophilus*) or *Bifidobacterium bifidum* to replenish the body with good bacteria. Lactic acid bacteria are often called *probiotics* and serve to maintain the health of the intestinal tract by producing acids and other compounds that inhibit the growth of disease-causing bacteria.

When to Call the Doctor: Food poisoning can be serious, especially for infants, young children, pregnant women, those with compromised immune systems, and older people, but call your doctor immediately—*regardless* of your Risk Quotient—if symptoms last longer than 24 hours, if you have blood in your stools, or if you cannot keep liquids down. If left untreated, some types of food poisoning can lead to liver damage and even death. Hepatitis A can cause similar symptoms, and your physician may wish to rule out this condition.

In addition, your physician may need to contact the local health department about a food poisoning outbreak and in doing so may learn that the causative agent has already been identified. *Save and label the food you have eaten* so it can be tested for specific pathogens to confirm the diagnosis, but make sure it is not accessible to anyone to consume.

Gingivitis

What Is It? Gingivitis is one of the most common forms of gum (periodontal) disease, affecting the tissues that support your teeth. It affects more than 75 percent of adults after age 35. However, there are many steps you can take to prevent gum disease and subsequent tooth loss.

What Causes It? Gum disease is caused by plaque, a sticky, colorless film of bacteria that coats your teeth, and the bacteria it contains. If allowed to harden, the film turns into tartar. This tartar irritates your gums, causing bleeding and swelling, and can lead to more serious gum disease (periodontitis) and eventually tooth loss.

Signs and Symptoms: With gingivitis, you can have a host of symptoms ranging from swollen or recessed gums, a sour or metallic taste in your mouth, bad breath, pain in one of your teeth when eating hot, cold, or sweet foods, loose teeth, or drainage or pus around one or more teeth.

Prevention and Treatment:

RQ 1 **Brush and floss your teeth regularly.** Use a fluoride toothpaste and brush thoroughly at least twice a day and after eating. Regular flossing each day can also help to prevent tartar buildup between your teeth as it cleans and stimulates the gums. Flossing is one self-care technique that can greatly reduce your chances of developing serious gingivitis.

See your dentist twice a year. A thorough cleaning by your dental hygienist rids your teeth of tartar and plaque. Cleaning also eliminates the source of irritation for your gums and stimulates them to heal.

Use an antiseptic mouthwash. Daily use of an over-the-counter mouthwash like Listerine or one that contains common thyme (*Thymus vulgaris*) reduces the bacteria in your mouth.

Chew sugar-free gum. Chewing gum helps to remove food particles from your teeth, plus it provides a bone-building workout—similar to the strengthening of bone that occurs when you lift weights at the gym.

Put these under your tongue. Both a sublingual coenzyme Q_{10} (CoQ_{10}) or a sublingual vitamin B_{12}/folic acid tablet can help healing.

RQ 2 **Watch your medications.** Some medications, such as antihistamines, can make you more susceptible to dry mouth, resulting in a buildup of bacteria. Talk to your doctor or dentist to see if this affects you.

Avoid snacking. Sticky or sweet snacks cause a buildup of bacteria if you do not clean your teeth immediately afterwards. It's best to avoid snacking if you are unable to brush.

RQ 3 **Get the right toothbrush.** Even with all the various textures of toothbrushes available, it's best to select one with soft, end-rounded or polished bristles. Make sure the brush is small enough to clean your back teeth as well as your front teeth, and replace your toothbrush with a new one after a month or two.

RQ 4 **Stop smoking.** Smoking is another contributing factor to gingivitis. Talk to your doctor about a smoking cessation program.

When to Call the Dentist: If your gums are swollen, bleed easily, and are deep red rather than pink in color, it's time to call your dentist. The earlier you see your dentist for an evaluation and cleaning, the greater your chances of keeping your gums and teeth healthy. Although uncertain, there might be a link between periodontal disease and a greater risk of heart attack or stroke—even more of a reason to brush, floss, and see your dentist regularly to prevent these serious health concerns.

Impetigo

What Is It? Although impetigo is a common childhood bacterial infection, it affects adults as well. This skin infection can occur just about anywhere on the body, but it is usually found around the buttocks, arms, mouth, or nose. It is highly contagious.

What Causes It? Blame the bacteria *Streptococcus* (strep) or *Staphylococcus* (staph) for most causes of mild impetigo. When your skin is irritated from scratching or from blowing your nose because of persistent allergic rhinitis, the bacteria congregate in that moist place and begin to multiply.

Signs and Symptoms: You may notice small red spots that look like tiny pimples. These spots may become itchy and quickly turn into blisters that burst open and secrete a sticky honey-colored substance. Sometimes a yellow crust can form on top of the impetigo. These circular spots can grow as large as a quarter.

Prevention and Treatment:

RQ 1 **Keep it clean.** Using a tissue or cotton ball, wash the infected area of skin several times each day with an antibacterial soap and warm water. Cover the impetigo sores with moist or wet gauze bandages after cleaning, even those sores on the face, if possible. Throw the tissue or cotton ball and old bandages away after cleaning, and wash your hands thoroughly.

Minimize contagion. Chances of impetigo spreading to other family members or friends are minimal if you wash your hands frequently and avoid touching the infection.

Consider a topical antibiotic. Sometimes your doctor will have to prescribe a topical antibiotic that is applied to the infection. Bactroban is one prescription antibacterial cream that's commonly used and may resolve most mild cases of impetigo.

RQ 2 **Keep skin healthy.** It's important to know that bacteria do not usually penetrate unbroken skin. You can help to prevent skin irritation by cleaning all wounds with soap and water. Keep open wounds covered, and put antibacterial ointment on wounded skin, if needed.

RQ 3 **Prevent infections.** Wash your sheets, clothes, and towels separately during the infection to prevent other family members from catching the impetigo.

RQ 4 Work with your doctor.

When to Call the Doctor: If the impetigo is spreading to different parts of your body or if it is worsening after 3 days of treatment with increased itching and oozing secretions, check with your doctor to see if antibiotics are needed. Impetigo is contagious.

Rosacea

What Is It? Rosacea is a common acnelike skin disease that affects the middle part of the face. More than 10 million adults have rosacea. Once rosacea develops in the skin, it lasts for years and usually does not reverse itself untreated.

What Causes It? While the cause of rosacea is unknown, it is thought that the condition may be related to the bacteria *Helicobacter pylori* (related to gastrointestinal ulcers), too little stomach acid, a mite found in the hair follicles, or as a result of vasodilators (medications taken for hypertension).

Signs and Symptoms: With this inflammation of the skin, tiny blood vessels in the middle third of the face (forehead, nose, chin) enlarge and become more pronounced through the skin. These vessels appear in this area like thin red lines. Sometimes pimples occur in rosacea, causing the skin condition to be mistaken for acne. Your skin will appear swollen and red—in fact, it looks as if you are blushing. If left untreated, rosacea can lead to rhinophyma, a disfiguring nose condition that literally causes the nose to grow (like W. C. Fields). If the eyes are involved, they may feel gritty and burn, which, in more serious cases, can lead to rosacea keratitis, a condition that damages the cornea and hinders vision.

Prevention and Treatment:

RQ 1 **Avoid the sun.** The sun aggravates rosacea, so wear a broad-brimmed hat and sunglasses when you are outdoors. Try sunscreen if it does not cause further irritation.

Use alcohol-free facial products. Cleanse your face with the mildest products that are made for sensitive skin. Avoid fragrances, powders, foundations, cheek blush, or any product that may cause the condition to flare.

RQ 2 **Watch your diet.** Rosacea may have many dietary triggers, including hot beverages, alcohol, caffeine, and spicy foods.

Meditate. Stress is another known trigger of rosacea. Take

10-minute time-outs throughout your day to meditate and reduce stress.

RQ 3 **Try vitamin E oil.** Dab a bit of pure, fragrance-free vitamin E oil (either bottled or from a vitamin E capsule) and see how your skin reacts. Some people find this is soothing to the inflamed skin, while others find it makes the skin too oily.

RQ 4 **Take a healing herbal combo.** Try the herbs echinacea (*Echinacea purpurea* or *E. angustifolia*), garlic (*Allium sativum*), and goldenseal (*Hydrastis canadensis*)—all known to have an antimi-

Promote Well-Being with Oils

Aromatherapists believe that essential oils have specific effects on mood and well-being. To try these oils for yourself and see if they work for you, add up to three drops of the oil to a carrier oil (olive, sesame, or another vegetable-based oil) for a soothing massage. Or put one or two drops on a candle's melted wax, and inhale the scent as the wax hardens. Don't use the oils while pregnant or nursing, and do not ingest them unless directed to do so under medical supervision. Store the oils in a cool, dark place.

Effect	Essential Oil
Increases mental alertness	Basil (*Ocimum basilicum*) Rosemary* (*Rosmarinus officinalis*) Lemon (*Citrus limon*)
Relieves insomnia	Lavender (*Lavandula angustifolia*) German chamomile (*Matricaria recutita*)
Improves sex drive	Sandalwood (*Santalum album*) Geranium (*Pelargonium graveolens*)
Soothes raw nerves	Frankincense (*Boswellia carteri*) Marjoram (*Origanum marjorana*)
Increases well-being	Jasmine (*Jasminum officinale*) Rose (*Rosa* spp.)

crobial and anti-inflammatory effect in the body. Echinacea may help fight both viral and bacterial infections, although how it does this is not yet fully understood.

When to Call the Doctor: See a doctor, specifically a dermatologist, for an accurate diagnosis and treatment. Rosacea is a chronic inflammatory skin condition that can grow worse—to the point where antibiotics are needed. Early diagnosis and treatment may prevent it from worsening and causing more serious problems.

Effect	Essential Oil
Decreases appetite	Dill (*Anethum graveolens*) Ginger (*Zingiber officinale*) Lemon (*Citrus limon*) Spearmint (*Mentha spicata*)
Relieves stress	Lavender (*Lavandula angustifolia*) Vanilla (*Vanilla planifolia*) German chamomile (*Matricaria recutita*)
Combats depression	Basil (*Ocimum basilicum*) Geranium (*Pelargonium graveolens*) Sweet orange (*Citrus sinensis*)
Boosts creativity	Peppermint** (*Mentha piperita*) Geranium (*Pelargonium graveolens*)
Increases energy	Sweet orange (*Citrus sinensis*) Peppermint** (*Mentha piperita*) Rosemary* (*Rosmarinus officinalis*)
Relieves PMS and cramps	Lavender (*Lavandula angustifolia*) German chamomile (*Matricaria recutita*)

*Do not use if you have hypertension or epilepsy, due to the powerful action on the nervous system.
**If you have gallbladder or liver disease, check with your doctor before using.

Sinus Infections

What Is It? Sinusitis is inflammation of the facial cavities around your nose—those above your eyes (frontal), behind the nose (sphenoids), on either side of the nose (ethmoid), and beneath the eyes in the cheek area (maxillary). They produce mucus, which drains through the ostia (small openings in the nose that allow your sinuses to drain). If the sinus cavities get clogged with mucus and the openings are blocked, infection and pain can result.

What Causes It? When conditions in the nose are healthy, the mucus is pushed out of your nose by cilia, which are tiny hairs that wave rhythmically to carry anything on their surface in the direction of their motion out of the respiratory tract. When conditions in the nose are not healthy, the cilia slow down or stop working properly, resulting in sinusitis. Or sinusitis can occur when there is an anatomical blockage, such as a deviated septum, and the stagnant mucus becomes infected. Some common causes of sinusitis include bacterial infections, cold viruses, allergic rhinitis, deviated septum, smoke, air pollution, and dry or cold air.

Signs and Symptoms: While many people suffer with sinusitis year-round, it is more common during the winter months and may be acute, chronic, or allergic fungal.

Acute sinusitis is usually caused by a bacterial infection or cold virus. It's important to treat acute sinusitis immediately to prevent other, more serious problems such as scarring in the sinuses. With acute sinusitis, you may have facial pressure, cold symptoms lasting for more than 10 days, green/yellow nasal discharge, a high fever (above 101° F), pain in your upper molars, and cough.

Chronic sinusitis feels like an ongoing cold—your nose keeps running and running. It is defined as an inflammation of the sinuses persisting more than 8 to 12 weeks and can occur for many reasons, including a bacterial infection. But chronic sinusitis usually occurs because the drainage passage from the sinuses to the nose becomes blocked. It is most often a chronic inflammatory disorder, similar to chronic bronchitis.

With chronic sinusitis, you harbor fewer symptoms than with acute sinusitis. You may just have a chronic sore throat and cough, particularly when reclining, and a decreased sense of smell. Or you may have nasal congestion and a low-grade fever (less than 101° F). Sometimes you may have drainage, sore throat, or a cough that lasts for days or even weeks. These annoying symptoms interfere with restful sleep.

Allergic fungal sinusitis (AFS) is just making medical news; it's the type of sinusitis scientists know the least about. In a study published in a 1999 issue of *Mayo Clinic Proceedings*, researchers examined 210 patients and found fungi in 96 percent of the patients' mucus. Although the fungus was prevalent in this study, allergic reaction to the fungus was suspected in only 10 percent of the patients. Most of us don't have this problem, but it's noteworthy.

Prevention and Treatment:

RQ 1

Massage the pain away. Massaging your sinuses brings a fresh blood supply to the area and soothing relief. Try pressing your thumbs firmly on both sides of your nose and hold for 10 to 20 seconds. (Don't press too hard on your face or neck, as you may damage delicate nerves, resulting in more pain than you had before!)

Liquefy the mucus. Drink at least 8 glasses (64 ounces) of water or clear liquid each day to hydrate the body and dilute the mucus.

RQ 2 **Reduce triggers.** There are a host of sinusitis triggers—pollen, dust, mold, pet dander, and chemicals—that can cause irritation. If you know what triggers your sinusitis, avoid it. Window air conditioner units should be cleaned annually and the same goes for central air vents in your house. Both can harbor molds and fungi, which can serve as triggers. Homes that have indoor pets should consider cleaning these units and vents more frequently.

Use moist heat. Many people get excellent relief by applying warm, moist compresses to the sinus area to increase drainage.

Try an herbal boost. Try supplementing with the herbs echinacea (*Echinacea purpurea* or *E. angustifolia*), garlic (*Allium sativum*), and goldenseal (*Hydrastis canadensis*)—all immune system stimulants that boost the body's natural defenses. In addition, freeze-dried nettle (*Urtica dioica*), quercetin, and vitamin C may help.

Decrease inflammation naturally. Another remedy to speed healing is drinking pineapple juice, which is rich in an enzyme called bromelain that helps the body to fight infection. You can also try bromelain tablets, which are available at most natural foods stores.

RQ 3 **Use hydrotherapy.** This is the use of water in all forms—from ice to steam—to promote healing. This complementary treatment works by stimulating your body's own healing force. Cold compresses reduce swelling by constricting blood vessels. (In fact, this is an excellent way to stop a nosebleed associated with sinusitis.) Conversely, warm, moist compresses on the sinus area can reduce the soreness and pain by increasing blood flow in and drainage out—an effective alternative treatment for sinus headache pain or congestion.

Sip tepid tea. Drink room temperature tea with no caffeine—and a lot of it. But avoid cold or iced drinks, as the cold temperature stops the cilia from functioning normally, causing the mucus to stagnate in the sinus passages. Water keeps your respiratory system hydrated, which helps to liquefy thick mucus that builds up to cause infection in your sinus cavity.

Take thyme. The immune-boosting herb thyme (*Thymus vulgaris*) contains the phytochemical thymol and has antitussive (anti-cough), antispasmodic, and expectorant properties. Common thyme is an ingredient in some antiseptic mouthwashes, throat lozenges, and herbal cough remedies. It is also used in herbal teas, especially for treating mild symptoms associated with coughs, bronchitis, or colds.

RQ 4 **Use a mucus mobilizer.** Try the over-the-counter medication guaifenesin, the main ingredient in Robitussin, known to liquefy mucus and help it to flow. When mucus is flowing, there is less chance of infection.

Avoid saltwater gargles. While swishing warm salt water in your mouth may help reduce throat pain, harsh gargling causes the uvula (the soft structure hanging in the back of your throat) to swell, which can increase the pain and inflammation.

Chew aspirin gum. Any flavor of this analgesic, such as Aspergum, works by numbing the tissue in the throat and helping to decrease inflammation, resulting in less pain. (But don't give this gum to your children because of the risk of Reye's syndrome. See page 213.)

Try antacids. Some people notice thickened mucus, postnasal drip, and other sinus symptoms as a result of gastroesophageal reflux disease (GERD). If your symptoms are caused by reflux, work to calm the acid. Sleeping on two pillows or elevating the head of your bed may also reduce the chance of irritation.

Boost immune power. Many people find relief with echinacea (*Echinacea purpurea* or *E. angustifolia*), an herbal supplement that has been shown in preliminary studies to boost immune function. Echinacea stimulates the production of interferon, a natural body substance important for the body's defense against disease. It has been found to increase levels of properdin, a natural compound that helps to destroy viruses, fungi, bacteria, and other disease-causing microbes. It may take a week before you notice a difference.

When to Call the Doctor: If your sinus symptoms are acute, ongoing, or worsen, call your doctor for an evaluation. A nasal smear may need to be cultured. Using a microscope, a doctor will view the culture, identify the bacteria, and then prescribe the necessary antibiotic to treat it. Your doctor may also instruct you on how to use saline nasal irrigation at home to continue drainage and prescribe antibiotics and decongestants for continued healing.

Sore Throat

What Is It? A sore throat is a real "pain in the neck" that sends nearly 40 million adults to the doctor's office each year for diagnosis and treatment. Whether from constant postnasal drip, swelling from inflamed tissue, or an all-out throat infection, sore throats can diminish your quality of life and productivity. As with the other bacteria-related infections, early self-care may help you avoid further problems and boost your resistance so the sore throat can resolve quickly.

What Causes It? When bacteria settle in your nose, they are seized and dragged off to the lymph glands where the good white cells are kept. More good blood comes to that area. There, the concentration of white cells can overwhelm the bacteria. But when the lymph material swells, this causes the painful throat you feel.

This throat infection may be bacterial or viral. The most important difference between bacteria and viruses is that bacteria respond well to antibiotic treatment, but viruses do not. Some of the most common causes of sore throat are:

- Sinus drainage
- Tonsillitis
- Gastroesophageal reflux disease (GERD), a condition resulting in intense heartburn
- Swollen uvula
- Mono (infectious mononucleosis)
- Strep
- Epiglottitis, a bacterial infection that causes the tissue at the back of the throat to become swollen, potentially closing the airway.

Signs and Symptoms: Your throat will feel swollen, scratchy, and raw. You may have difficulty swallowing without pain. If the lower one-third of the throat is infected, you may be hoarse because your larynx is swollen and cannot function properly. Consult your doctor if you have very large, swollen tonsils with a white coating and red or white spots, swollen and tender neck glands, headache, nausea, or a fine rash (scarlet fever, which indicates strep throat).

Prevention and Treatment:

RQ 1 **Stay hydrated.** Drink copious amounts of water. Drink a minimum of 8 glasses (64 ounces) of water per day when afflicted with a sore throat.

RQ 2 **Drink herbal tea.** Ginger (*Zingiber officinale*) tea can be particularly soothing.

RQ 3 **Try zinc lozenges.** Sucking on zinc lozenges (especially zinc-gluconate with glycine) at the start of a sore throat may lessen its severity. The body may be unable to fight infection without sufficient supplies of this nutrient.

Use analgesics. To numb the pain, you can use aspirin, acetaminophen (Tylenol), or a nonsteroidal anti-inflammatory drug (NSAID) like ibuprofen (Advil). If you cannot take these pain relievers, check with your doctor about another option to reduce pain.

Avoid dairy foods. While dairy foods may not cause your sore throat, some people find that they coat the back of the throat, making it feel more inflamed than it already is. Once the condition is resolved, introduce dairy again. Similarly, bananas, oranges, and peanuts may contribute to mucus production, so you might also try to avoid them until you're feeling better.

RQ 4 **Avoid known irritants.** Avoid smoking and pollutant exposure as well as any food allergens. Gentle gargling with acidophilus (*Lactobacillus acidophilus*), beneficial bacteria that compete with the harmful ones, can prove helpful.

Run the humidifier. If the air is dry, a cool mist humidifier or vaporizer can moisten the air and make it easier to breathe. Keep the humidifier clean, however, to prevent the growth of bacteria, molds, and fungi.

Try mullein. The herb mullein (*Verbascum thapsus*) contains the active constituents mucilage, saponins, and tannins, which help to soothe mucous membranes and a scratchy throat and have antibacterial action. It also calms the bronchial muscle spasm that causes the constant coughing. Try mullein tea—it's bitter in taste, so add honey to sweeten.

When to Call the Doctor: If you suspect strep, mono, or epiglottitis, call your doctor immediately. Strep infection usually needs treatment with antibiotics because of rare complications such as rheumatic fever (which can lead to heart damage) or poststreptococcal glomerulonephritis (a kidney complication where blood and protein are detected in the urine). A blood test is necessary to diagnose mono, and treatment is limited. Reduce activities that may result in abdominal trauma, since mono can cause enlargement of the spleen, which can rupture, causing potentially catastrophic consequences. With epiglottitis, the most serious type of throat infection, a bacteria targets part of the voice box (larynx), resulting in inflammation or swelling that actually closes the airway. You may have difficulty swallowing or speaking, and breathing will become labored. Emergency medical attention is necessary if this happens.

Sty

What Is It? A sty is a relatively common bacterial infection that usually develops near the root (follicle) of the eyelash. It looks and feels like a pimple, as it is red and filled with pus. Sties usually start and resolve within 1 or 2 days.

What Causes It? Sties result when bacteria build up inside of the follicle of an eyelash. You may have more than one sty at a time or several in succession.

Signs and Symptoms: A sty starts as an itchy or painful swelling on the eyelid. Your eye will be red, and you will have tearing and blurred vision. It may feel as if something is under your eyelid, which will also be red, but usually there's no change in visual acuity.

Prevention and Treatment:

RQ 1 **Use warm compresses.** You can find good relief with applications of warm compresses for 5 minutes, several times a day, which help to decrease pain and increase healing. When the sty comes to a head and bursts on its own, clean your eye with damp cotton balls and throw them away to avoid reinfection.

Wash hands. Although sties are not thought to be contagious, make sure you wash your hands frequently throughout the day and use paper towels to prevent the infection from spreading to others.

RQ 2 **Use saline drops.** You can purchase saline eye drops without antihistamines over-the-counter. Use these frequently to keep your eye moist. Once the sty has popped, throw the eye drops away to keep bacteria from reinfecting you or other family members.

RQ 3 **Try hydrotherapy.** If moist heat applications do not alleviate swelling, alternate applications of warm and cold washcloths, using 5 minutes of warm followed by 1 minute of cold. Do this alternate application three times each every few hours.

RQ 4 **"B" smart.** Add a vitamin B complex. The B vitamins are essential for maintaining healthy skin.

Get herbal relief. Try bromelain, the healing enzyme in pineapple, which can offer anti-inflammatory relief when taken internally. As noted in a 2001 study, bromelain may help to speed wound healing, reducing pain, tenderness, and swelling. You can find bromelain tablets at most natural foods stores.

When to Call the Doctor: If the sty continues to remain swollen after a few days or is painful and affecting your vision, call your doctor to see whether it needs to be lanced to drain the infection. Seek immediate medical attention with any change in visual acuity. Such changes can be caused by numerous ocular conditions such as detached retina or iritis.

Tonsillitis

What Is It? Tonsillitis occurs when the tonsils, the lymphatic tissues in the back of the throat, become infected.

What Causes It? In a healthy mouth, the tonsils help to prevent infection in the body by filtering out bacteria and other microorganisms. In some cases, usually when you are run down and have poor resistance to infection, the tonsils become overwhelmed by viral or bacterial infections. (Chronic tonsillitis can be a source of recurrent infection with strep or *Haemophilus influenzae*.)

Signs and Symptoms: With tonsillitis, you will have a sore, swollen throat. You may have difficulty swallowing because of the swelling. If you look at your tonsils with a mirror, they will appear red, swollen, and may be coated in white spots. You may also have a fever and feel fatigued and achy all over.

Prevention and Treatment:

RQ 1 **Get more rest.** Getting plenty of rest and sleep is important to boost immune function and give the body time to heal. It is during the deeper stages of sleep that the healing process works best.

Drink additional water. Your tonsils act as filters for foreign invaders. Keeping your body well-hydrated helps tonsils to function optimally and helps to prevent their congestion.

RQ 2 **Take an analgesic.** Ibuprofen (Advil) or acetaminophen (Tylenol) both work well to resolve the pain of tonsillitis.

Use papain. These natural papaya enzyme tablets can ease inflammation in the throat. They are easily absorbed into the body if taken dissolved in your mouth between your cheek and gums.

RQ 3 RQ 4 **Gargle gently with warm salt water.** While vigorous gargling may injure the inflamed tissue in the throat, gently swishing warm salt water around and spitting it out may help alleviate the pain and scratchiness of tonsillitis.

Suck on zinc lozenges. Zinc (especially zinc-gluconate with glycine) may help boost immunity. The body may be unable to fight infection without sufficient supplies of this nutrient, and people deficient in zinc should consider eating more zinc-rich foods or supplementing. See "Dietary Reference Intakes" on page 164.

When to Call the Doctor: If the tonsillitis worsens with increased or persistent pain, if you cannot swallow or have difficulty breathing, or if your fever spikes higher than 101° F, call your doctor right away. You may have a bacterial infection that needs medical treatment.

Tooth Decay

What Is It? Tooth decay is a very common disease that affects all ages alike. The decay slowly eats away at the tooth, resulting in cavities. When tooth decay is left untreated, it can become severe enough to destroy the internal structures of the tooth and eventually end up in tooth loss.

What Causes It? In a healthy mouth, bacteria are normally present to convert all foods into acids. When the bacteria, acid, saliva, and food combine in the mouth, a sticky substance called plaque is formed that adheres to the teeth. Plaque is most noticeable on the molars, where there are uneven or grooved surfaces. It is also at the edge of the gum line and around fillings. The acids in plaque cause cavities. When these holes become large and deep, they can cause the nerves and blood vessels in the tooth to die (tooth abscess). When plaque is not removed, it mineralizes and turns into tartar. Together, plaque and tartar cause more damage, irritating the gums and resulting in gingivitis (gum disease).

Signs and Symptoms: With tooth decay, you may see holes or discolorations in your teeth. If left untreated, you may have tooth sensitivity to hot, cold, or sweet foods, and tooth pain. When tooth decay results in a tooth abscess, you may have redness or swelling in the gum over the tooth and pain that can extend from the tooth into the jaw and ear (referred pain).

Prevention and Treatment:

RQ 1 **Practice prevention.** Brush your teeth at least twice a day with a soft brush and fluoride toothpaste. Floss between your teeth at least once a day.

RQ 2 **Minimize snacking.** Snacking keeps your mouth acidic, which can encourage tooth decay. Instead of eating sugary, chewy, or sticky foods, chew sugar-free gum if you have the urge to snack. Drink water and unsweetened beverages.

RQ 3 **Ask about a fluoride rinse or sealants.** If you are prone to tooth decay and the resulting cavities, ask your dentist whether a fluoride rinse may help to prevent further problems. These are available over-the-counter at most grocery and drug stores. Also ask your dentist about sealants, plastic films that are applied to the surface of teeth to seal off the pits and grooves where food and bacteria can be trapped and cause decay.

RQ 4 **Boost your calcium intake.** Keep your teeth, gums, and bones strong by increasing foods rich in calcium, including dairy products (milk, cheeses, yogurt, and ice cream), greens (mustard, kale, and turnip), okra, oranges, salmon (canned with bones), sardines (canned with bones), tofu (processed with calcium sulfate) and other soy products, and other calcium-enriched foods.

Consider coronation. A crown (covering) is useful if your tooth has large cavities or multiple fillings. The porcelain or gold material is shaped to fit your tooth and keeps it from further decay or breaking.

When to Call the Dentist: Seeing your dentist at least twice a year for a professional exam and cleaning is important. If you have any signs of tooth decay, including pain, sensitivity, or holes in the teeth, then make an appointment immediately to get the problem treated. Early treatment of tooth decay can stop the damage and save the tooth. If you delay treatment, you may suffer needlessly, both physically and financially.

Ulcers

What Is It? An ulcer is a sore or an area of raw tissue in the stomach (gastric ulcers) or in the part of the intestine that drains food from the stomach (duodenal ulcers).

What Causes It? More than 90 percent of all ulcers are caused by a bacterium, *Helicobacter pylori*, that adheres to the cells in the lining of the stomach and causes tissue damage. Other causes include excessive stomach acidity, anti-inflammatory drugs (aspirin, ibuprofen), inflammation, and irritation. Ulcer pain is usually worst between meals and at night when the stomach is empty, as acid irritates the stomach cells.

Signs and Symptoms: Symptoms of an ulcer include burning, belching, and bloating in the stomach, gas, nausea, and blood in the stool.

Prevention and Treatment:

RQ 1 **Avoid irritants.** Smoking, alcohol, caffeine, chocolate, fried or spicy foods, and nuts are often associated with ulcers, as they irritate the lining of the stomach and increase acid production.

RQ 2 **Identify the cause.** Many ulcers these days are believed to be caused by *H. pylori*, which can be easily tested for. If the cause is *H. Pylori*, then it warrants specific treatment.

RQ 3 **De-stress.** While scientists are not sure of the exact cause of ulcers, it's thought that stress plays a role, in that it may increase the production of acid, which can irritate the stomach lining. Make sure you allow for downtime throughout your day to reflect on the moment—and not your worries and problems.

Eat cabbage. There is now evidence that raw cabbage juice, a folk remedy, may kill *H. pylori* without exposing you to antibiotic overuse. Cabbage and its juice contain large amounts of glutamine and S-methylmethionine, two compounds with anti-ulcer activity. In clinical studies, researchers found 92 percent of those who drank raw cabbage juice had significant improvement in ulcer symptoms in just 3 weeks. You need to ingest 1 quart of the raw cabbage juice daily for optimal benefit, but it can be used in vegetable soups to make it more palatable.

RQ 4 **Boost immune function.** Try supplementing with the herbs echinacea (*Echinacea purpurea* or *E. angustifolia*), garlic (*Allium sativum*), and goldenseal (*Hydrastis canadensis*)—all known to have an antimicrobial and anti-inflammatory affect in the body. Echinacea may help fight both viral and bacterial infections, although how it does this is not fully understood. If you are sensitive to fresh garlic, consider supplements.

Get relief. Deglycyrrhizinised licorice (DGL) has been shown to be as effective in the long-term treatment of ulcers as Tagamet, an over-the-counter heartburn relief medication. Other nonprescription remedies include Pepcid AC, Zantac 75, and Axid AR; these are low-dose versions of prescription H2 blockers, drugs that inhibit the production of stomach acids. Temporary relief can also be provided by antacid tablets, which neutralize acid. If you take an H2 blocker or an over-the-counter remedy, ask your doctor about trying DGL while you taper off those medications. Or ask your doctor about slippery elm (*Ulmus rubra*) or marshmallow leaf (*Althaea officinalis*), both of which have a coating effect on the digestive tract and can provide relief.

When to Call the Doctor: Ulcers can be serious. If your symptoms are acute (sudden) or persist, call your doctor for an evaluation. If you cough up blood or have black stools or blood in the stools, feel light-headed, or have nausea or vomiting, this could signal a more serious problem that needs immediate medical attention.

Urinary Tract Infections

What Is It? A urinary tract infection (UTI) is a common but serious infection that can affect the kidneys, ureter, bladder, and urethra. Each year more than eight million Americans are affected by UTIs, with one woman in five experiencing a UTI in her lifetime.

What Causes It? In a healthy environment, most urine is sterile. However, in some cases, microorganisms, usually bacteria from the digestive tract, adhere to the opening of the urethra and start to reproduce and multiply. Most of the time, UTIs are caused by *Escherichia coli* (*E. coli*) bacteria, which live in the colon but can enter the urinary tract during sexual intercourse or by wiping from back to front.

Bacteria usually start reproducing in the urethra. If the infection is self-contained in the urethra, it's called urethritis. When the infection spreads, it may move to the bladder (cystitis; see "Bladder Infections [Cystitis]" on page 93) or go up the ureter to the kidneys (pyelonephritis).

While some people are more prone to getting a UTI, anytime there is an obstruction in the natural flow of urine—for example, a kidney stone or an enlarged prostate gland—this infection is possible. People who have diabetes or challenged immune systems are also more prone to UTIs.

nd Symptoms: With a urinary tract infection, you may ure above the pelvic bone (for women) or in the rectum (for inful urination, and experience frequency in urination and cl urine, although some people have no symptoms at all. Sometimes ou might find it difficult to pass more than a few drops of urine, even though you have a tremendous urge to urinate. If the UTI involves the kidneys, you may run a fever and have pain in the back or side (below your ribs), along with feelings of nausea and vomiting.

Prevention and Treatment:

RQ 1 **Address the problem.** Urinary tract infections can be caused by a host of problems—from bubble baths, scented tissue, and other local irritants to vaginal tissue changes or benign prostate problems. Figure out what is causing your problem, and make changes to remove the offenders.

Stay hydrated. Drink 8 glasses (64 ounces) of water daily to help the urine stay diluted and to encourage kidney function.

Urinate frequently. Urinate frequently throughout the day and immediately after intercourse to help prevent urine from becoming stagnant.

RQ 2

Use the rules of good hygiene. You can avoid getting a UTI if you follow the rules of good hygiene. For women, make sure you avoid fecal contamination by wiping from the front to the back after going to the bathroom. Avoid synthetic underwear and nylon stockings, both of which can trap moisture. Avoid bubble baths, which can contribute to UTIs, and make sure your sexual partner practices good hygiene, as well.

Stay moist. Make sure vaginal tissues stay moist and avoid irritation that could cause swelling, making it difficult to urinate.

Eliminate diuretics. Eliminate caffeine and other diuretics that can be dehydrating and increase pain and irritation. Talk with your doctor about this, particularly if you are on a constrained diet.

RQ 3

Drink unsweetened cranberry juice. Some studies show cranberry juice lowers *E. coli* adhesion, while other juices such as orange or grapefruit did not.

Avoid sugar. Eating too much sugar can decrease immune function, setting the stage for infection. Find other healthful snacks that are low in sugar, especially if you are prone to infection.

Increase antioxidants. Add daily supplements of vitamin C to protect against infection and to aid in tissue healing. Vitamin C is a major player in helping the body from the formation of free radicals. Free radicals cause damage to the cells and impair the immune system. When you add vitamin C supplementation or boost your intake of vitamin C (and other antioxidants), you can increase the free radical scavenging process.

RQ 4 **Try herbal therapy.** The herb uva-ursi (*Arctostaphylos uva-ursi*) helps to soothe, tone, and strengthen the membranes of the urinary system. The active ingredient in uva-ursi is glycoside arbutin, which has been shown to kill bacteria in the urine. Also try buchu (*Barosma betulina*), an herb that acts as an antiseptic to the urinary tract system. Both uva-ursi and buchu can be found at natural foods stores.

Boost healing with essential nutrients. Take essential fatty acids (EFAs), such as fish oil, flaxseed oil, evening primrose oil (*Oenothera biennis*), or borage oil (*Borago officinalis*), and vitamin E to help boost tissue healing.

Add zinc. Zinc has tremendous antioxidant effects and is vital to your body's resistance to infection and for tissue repair. Many illnesses, including kidney disease and long-term infection, are associated with zinc deficiency. If you are taking medication, it may interfere with zinc absorption in the intestines and cause a zinc deficiency. To improve immune function, eat foods high in zinc including seafood, eggs, meats, whole grains, wheat germ, nuts, and seeds; coffee and tea may hinder zinc absorption.

When to Call the Doctor: A urinary tract infection can be very serious. If you have difficulty urinating, blood in your urine, burning urination, pain in your lower back, or fever, call your doctor. If treated early, UTIs can be resolved quickly with antibiotics. However, if you wait to treat this common bacteria-related problem, kidney damage can result.

Vaginitis

What Is It? Vaginitis (vaginosis) is an increase in the amount of discharge, a change in the color or smell of the discharge, and irritation, itchiness, or burning in or around the vagina. Sometimes this discharge is stained with blood. To best treat vaginitis, it's important to first see your doctor for a diagnostic test to identify the infecting organism.

What Causes It? This female problem is caused by a host of organisms (fungal, bacterial, or the protozoa *Trichomonas vaginalis*, among others) or anything that upsets the normal balance in the vagina. Sometimes douching will lead to vaginitis, as can bath soaps, scented sprays, or bubble baths.

Candidiasis, or yeast infection, is a common fungal infection that happens when there is an abundance of the fungus *Candida albicans*. While this fungus is always present in the body, when an imbalance occurs, such as with hormonal changes, use of antibiotics, a disease such as diabetes, or when the normal acidity of the vagina changes, it can multiply. Candidiasis results in pruritus, an itching sensation that triggers the desire to scratch, along with a thick, white vaginal discharge, vaginal burning, or painful intercourse.

If you have bacterial vaginosis caused by *Gardnerella vaginalis* bacteria, it is not clear what causes this infection. Antibiotic therapy is the best treatment for this infection.

The organism *Trichomonas vaginalis* is another cause of vaginitis. This is usually caused by having unprotected sex with an infected partner. You may or may not have signs for a long time, and it is treated with antibiotics; failure to treat this infection can jeopardize your ability to have a baby.

Warfarin Warning

Always read the warning information on any medication. If you take the prescription blood-thinner warfarin (Coumadin) and have a vaginal yeast infection, for instance, check with your doctor before using an over-the-counter vaginal miconazole product. Miconazole, an anti-fungal drug, is available as creams and suppositories and has been available by prescription and over-the-counter for many years. While it is safely used in most women to treat yeast infections, the FDA issued a warning in March 2001 that it may cause abnormal blood clotting tests in women taking blood thinners. In addition to abnormal tests, one woman reported bruising, bleeding gums, and a nosebleed. The new FDA warning states: "Ask a doctor or pharmacist before use if you are taking the prescription blood-thinning medicine warfarin, because bleeding or bruising may occur."

Chlamydia and gonorrhea, two sexually transmitted infections of the cervix caused by bacteria, can also cause vaginal discharge and discomfort. These diseases must be treated with antibiotics.

Signs and Symptoms: With vaginitis you may notice a foul odor (particularly after sex or after bathing), a thick or discolored discharge (often gray, yellowish, or white), itchiness, burning upon urination, or inflammation.

Prevention and Treatment:

RQ 1

Stay well-hydrated. Drink at least 8 glasses (64 ounces) of water each day, to help protect your skin.

Stay moist. Keep the vaginal tissues moist. If there is insufficient lubrication during sexual intercourse, use a lubricant to avoid injuring tissues. (Always use water-based lubricants like K-Y Jelly rather

Dietary Reference Intakes

	Calcium (mg/day)	Vit B_6 (mg/day)	Vit B_{12} (mcg/day)	Vit C (mg/day)	Vit E (mg/day)	Zinc (mg/day)	Selenium (mcg/day)
Boys							
9–13	1,300	1.0	1.8	45	11	8	40
14–18	1,300	1.3	2.4	75	15	11	55
Girls							
9–13	1,300	1.0	1.8	45	11	8	40
14–18	1,300	1.2	2.4	65	15	9	55
Men							
19–30	1,000	1.3	2.4	90	15	11	55
31–50	1,000	1.3	2.4	90	15	11	55
51–70	1,200	1.7	2.4	90	15	11	55
Women							
19–30	1,000	1.3	2.4	75	15	8	55
31–50	1,000	1.3	2.4	75	15	8	55
51–70	1,200	1.5	2.4	75	15	8	55

than petroleum-based products that don't work.) Some find relief with vitamin E suppositories to nourish tissue and help lubrication.

Avoid tight-fitting clothes. Tight pants or underwear can rub and irritate sensitive tissue. Wear loose-fitting clothes until the infection clears up.

RQ 2 **Use caution.** Use common sense when it comes to having sexual relations with individuals who have sexually transmitted diseases, always use a condom, and avoid undue friction during intercourse. Avoid douching, as this can irritate sensitive tissues.

Eat yogurt. The active bacterial cultures in yogurt may help to prevent vaginal yeast infections. Make sure the label on your yogurt says that it contains live cultures.

RQ 3 **Up your EFAs.** Essential fatty acids (EFAs) are not manufactured by the body but are essential to promote healing and are available in fish and flaxseed oils, which contain omega-3.

RQ 4 **Use nutritional therapy.** Make sure your diet includes plenty of whole foods high in antioxidants (vitamins A, C, and E) and zinc. (See "Dietary Reference Intakes," opposite, for more information on safe levels of some of these vitamins.)

When to Call the Doctor: There are many types of vaginal and vulvar problems that can cause the same symptoms as a yeast infection. For a correct diagnosis, a doctor should perform laboratory tests including microscopic evaluation of vaginal fluid. It is much wiser to get an accurate diagnosis and treat the problem correctly—and quickly—than to waste time with self-care that just won't work.

4

CARING FOR YOUR CHILDREN

Like you, I would go to the ends of the Earth to protect my children. As a parent, I work hard to provide nutritious meals, quality medical care, and an excellent education. Why, then, don't I call the pediatrician for antibiotics every time they complain of a sore throat or earache or run a fever? The reason is simple: The misuse or overuse of antibiotics is not good for kids. In fact, studies suggest that antibiotic overkill may lead to serious health problems in years to come.

Kids are clearly one group at a relatively high risk for infection. Not only do most of them spend hours every day in close contact with other children their age, whether in day care or crowded classrooms, but they also tend to practice poor hygiene. This puts pressure on their developing immune systems to do battle with a whole host of noxious germs that can result in symptoms such as fever, runny nose, cough, and diarrhea, among others. While antibiotics are usually necessary for bacterial illnesses, many common childhood illnesses are caused by viruses, including some respiratory and ear infections, and *antibiotics have no effect on viruses*. Yet Americans continue to believe that antibiotics are wonder drugs that can cure all. A study reported in *Pediatrics* documented that approximately half of a sample of pediatricians reported that parents pressured them to prescribe antibiotics for a sick child when, in the doctor's opinion, antibiotics were not indicated.

A perfect example of our love affair with antibiotics is the overuse in treating childhood acute otitis media (AOM), or middle ear infection, which is by far the most frequent use of antibiotics for young children. In recent years, doctors treated most childhood ear infections with a 10-day or 2-week course of antibiotics. If this failed to resolve the ear pain and fluid buildup, the child received a combination of stronger antibiotics or even long-term antibiotic therapy, taking these drugs for 3 or 4 months at a time. This was thought to be the gold standard of treatment, although a 2001 study published in the *Journal of the American Medical Association* suggested that shorter courses of treatment might be as effective.

In addition, some intriguing studies from countries around the world that do not use antibiotics as standard treatment are showing weak results that the use of antibiotics for otitis media decreases the severity of symptoms, and more than 80 percent of children with AOM get well within 1 to 7 days without antibiotics.

So where does this leave parents who want the best for their children yet who do not understand the problem of antibiotic resistance? Parents are often vulnerable as they face unreasonable pressure from child-care staff or classroom teachers to put their children on antibiotics for viral infections such as colds or sore throats. A revealing study presented at the International Conference on Emerging Infectious Disease in

2000, held in Atlanta, reported that very few day care workers knew that antibiotics would not end a cold more quickly or prevent it from spreading. The study showed that the majority of day care workers in the United States would allow children with colds to stay at day care, but only if they were taking antibiotics, a policy that promotes both the spreading of viral illnesses among children *and* antibiotic resistance. Children with colds who were not taking antibiotics often were sent home. Perhaps mass public awareness campaigns throughout the United States will get across the message of antibiotic resistance and offer some hope on the health horizon for our children.

The Hygiene Hypothesis

Most parents have always hoped that it's harmless for children to put food or a toy that they pick up off the floor into their mouths. There is now a new hypothesis that while early childhood infections are thought to have a protective effect against the development of asthma and allergies, the use of antibiotics at that vulnerable age may lead to an increased risk of these same illnesses. The Hygiene Hypothesis, mentioned briefly in chapter 1, is an emerging theory that came from repeated attempts to explain variances in asthma and allergy prevalence related to socioeconomic and geographic factors. It suggests that raising children in germ- and illness-free environments can compromise their immune systems.

Immune System Balancing

Whether it ultimately emerges as the prevailing theory, the Hygiene Hypothesis represents the "use it or lose it" concept with respect to the immune system. According to the Hygiene Hypothesis, our immune system is like a set of scales. When the scales are balanced, meaning routinely challenged but not overwhelmed, we are in optimal health. But when the scale is tipped far enough, it can result in declining health and chronic or life-threatening illness. For example, in a healthy body, one part of the immune system deploys white blood cells that assault infected cells; another part produces antibodies that block dangerous microbes from invading the body's cells in the first place. Some scientists now theorize that an imbalance can occur with the two parts of the immune system if it does not get stimulation during the early part of a child's life, either through fighting viruses and infections or through encounters with certain harmless microbes, such as mycobacteria found in dirt and untreated water (yes, sand castles and mud pies!). In fact, some believe the Hygiene Hypothesis is the basis for the skyrocketing number of childhood allergies, asthma, and other autoimmune diseases such as rheumatoid arthritis and Type 1 diabetes. I'm still unsure about

Common Allergens

FOOD
Corn
Dairy products
Peanuts
Soy
Wheat products

INDOOR
Aerosols
Cockroaches
Dander from pets
Dust
Dust mites
Feathers/Down
Fumes
Mold
Smoke
Wood-burning stoves
Wool

OUTDOOR
Dust
Environmental pollution
Grass
Industrial pollution
Mold spores
Pollen
Ragweed
Trees

this hypothesis, and it requires a great deal more investigation. A variety of other social changes may also explain the observed increases: fewer parents stay at home to cook and clean, so children may actually be exposed to indoor environments that are not as clean; smoking rates among women have increased; a larger number of households now have indoor pets; and today's homes have become more airtight.

Day Care Data

Some surprising scientific studies have shown that children who were around other children, whether in large families or in day care, had fewer allergies than children who were in small families or who did not attend day care. In one fascinating study published in 2000 in the *New England Journal of Medicine*, scientists at the University of Arizona followed a group of children from infancy until age 13. In babies under 6 months, those who were in day care or who had older siblings had higher rates of illness, including asthma and wheezing. But by the time these children were 6 to 13 years old, they were 40 percent less likely to suffer from asthma. These findings imply that exposure of young children to older children at home or to other children at day care may give their immune systems a workout and help protect against the development of asthma later in childhood. This study is similar to one performed in Germany, reported in 1999 in *The Lancet*, in which the frequency of asthma in children 5 to 14 years old was lower among those who had begun attending day care early in life than among those who had been enrolled in day care later.

At the same time, in a 1998 study published in *Thorax*, researchers theorized that children who received oral antibiotics by age 2 were more susceptible to allergies than children who had no antibiotics. These results may indicate that antibiotic treatment, which depletes the harmless bacteria within the gut, derails early immune development. Some researchers believe that the overuse of antibiotics may also affect the gastrointestinal tract, leading to an increased incidence of food allergies. In a study published in 1999 in *The Lancet*, Swedish scientists concluded that children from families that avoid antibiotics and vaccinations have fewer allergies than other children do. (While I do find the scientific data on antibiotic overuse and atopic disease compelling, I believe that every child *must* be immunized; I discuss this later in the chapter.) As with many other studies, it is difficult to control for factors that might also explain the observations, so uncertainty remains.

A Little Dirt May Be Just What the Doctor Ordered

When I grew up, kids spent a lot of time playing outside in the dirt. I remember my brother and I playing outdoors with our friends most of the day. We often slept with the windows open during some times of the year, enjoying the cool night air. Today kids rarely play outside, either for safety issues or because many are glued to the television set or computer games. Except for organized sports, most children stay indoors, breathing recycled air in their well-insulated homes while their exposure to the outdoors and all the microorganisms living there is extremely limited. You have to wonder if this lifestyle habit is resulting in an increase of autoimmune diseases in addition to increasing obesity. Scientists just don't know.

I think it's important to introduce you to scientific theories like the Hygiene Hypothesis that try to make sense of serious public health problems. But keep in mind, this theory is untested and surrounded with controversy. Given the uncertainty, I believe the best advice is to focus on your family's Personal Health Risk Profiles, which I explained in chapter 2, and the multitude of hands-on tools detailed in chapters 3 through 7 to keep your child healthy and avoid overkill.

How Childhood Diseases Are Transmitted

While theories are fine to consider, let's talk realistically about our kids. Before I give you the four steps parents can take to keep their kids healthy, it's important to clearly understand how bacteria and viruses are transmitted. Once you know how the different types of germs are spread (and it does vary) and who is most susceptible to getting the germs, the proactive measures I suggest to keep your children well will make great sense.

For germs to spread from one person to another, three key things must happen:

1. Germs must be present. Either a person is carrying the germs; the germs are in the air or on a surface; or the germs are in body fluids such as mucus from the person's nose, a discharge from the eye, or saliva from the mouth.

2. A person who is not immune to the germs must come in contact with them. This could happen by touching a doorknob after a person with a cold had touched it, kissing someone who is sick, or being in the path of someone's uncontrolled sneeze.

3. This point of contact or exposure must happen in such a way that leads to infection. Thus, the nonimmune person must not only contact the germs but also must introduce them effectively into his body—either by touching parts of his face or by eating with unwashed hands so that the germs get inside his body, where they can begin to affect the new host.

Keep in mind that the hands are one of the biggest transporters of germs, and as a parent you know that kids touch everything in sight. Germs can be transmitted directly to others or indirectly through household objects that other family members are likely to touch after you. Remember, as I mentioned in chapter 1, infections are commonly spread through one of several routes, and the chart on page 178 shows you how some of the most common childhood diseases are spread.

Common Childhood Diseases and Pathogens

Refer to the chart that follows this list, on page 178, to see how common, disease-causing germs are transmitted.

Bacterial meningitis. A life-threatening inflammation of the meninges caused by a bacterial infection. The pathogens causing approximately 80 percent of cases include *Neisseria meningitides*, *Haemophilus influenzae*, and *Streptococcus pneumoniae*. Treatment involves powerful antibiotics and intravenous liquids to avoid dehydration. Vaccines are available against all three organisms. *H. influenzae* and *S. pneumoniae* vaccines are part of the standard childhood vaccination panel, and vaccination against *N. meningitides* is now recommended for college dorm residents.

Campylobacter. A leading cause of bacterial food poison that can result in inflammatory diarrhea, nausea, and fever. It is usually spread by eating or cross-contamination of contaminated poultry. Doctors use antibiotics to treat patients with *Campylobacter* food poisoning.

Chickenpox. A benign primary infection resulting in skin lesions and rash because of the varicella-zoster virus, a herpes virus. Chickenpox can be transferred by inhaling particle droplets exhaled when someone else talks, sneezes, or coughs or by touching the skin lesions. A vaccine is part of the standard childhood vaccination panel.

Cold. A common viral respiratory infection that causes sneezing, congestion, sore throat, and overall aches. There is no vaccine or cure.

Cold sores (fever blisters). Small sores on the mouth or lips caused by the herpes simplex type 1 virus. Commonly spread by kissing and other intimate contact, treatment is available to reduce pain, but there is no cure or vaccine.

Conjunctivitis. Inflammation of the membrane covering the eyeball that is caused by infection, irritation, or as the result of some systemic diseases such as chlamydial and gonococcal conjunctivitis or scleritis.

Cytomegalovirus. A common herpes virus that causes mononucleosis-like symptoms with fever and hepatitis (inflammation of the liver). This virus is spread through contact with saliva, urine, or other body fluids. While very dangerous during pregnancy, there is no vaccine or cure.

Diphtheria. A serious infection of the tonsils and upper respiratory tract that is transmitted the same way as a cold. A vaccine is part of the standard childhood vaccination panel (it's the "D" in DPT).

***E. coli* O157:H7.** A strain of *Escherichia coli* that, when ingested, produces toxins that can cause serious disease and death. Cases should be treated in a hospital with supportive care immediately. This particular strain causes severe diarrhea, often bloody, and lasts for a week or longer. There is no vaccine, and to date studies, like the one in the *New England Journal of Medicine*, suggest that antibiotic treatment may increase the risk of serious renal disease.

Enterovirus. A class of viruses, including poliovirus, coxsackievirus, and echovirus, that comes into the body through the gastrointestinal tract or respiratory system and may attack the nervous system, heart, lining of the lung or cause skin rash. There is no vaccine or cure for this class, but an experimental drug exists.

Fifth disease. Common in day care and dangerous to the fetus during pregnancy and caused by the human parvovirus B19, fifth disease causes a low-grade fever, malaise, a bright rash on the cheeks, and overall body rash. It is transmitted through droplets in the air, such as when someone infected with the disease sneezes or coughs, and there is no vaccine or cure.

***Haemophilus influenzae* type b (Hib).** An infection that causes fever and chills and is a leading cause of bacterial meningitis for young children, a serious condition that can result in mental retardation. A vaccine is part of the standard childhood vaccination panel, and with widespread vaccination of children in the United States, incidence of bacterial meningitis has dropped markedly.

Hand-foot-mouth disease. A syndrome caused by a variety of viruses that belong to a group called the enteroviruses. Hand-foot-mouth disease results in tiny blisters or a rash on the hands, feet, and the lining of the mouth.

Head lice. Parasitic insects that are found on the head and in hair. No vaccine exists, but treatment shampoos are available as well as special combs for removal of nits (lice larva). Periodic inspection of your child's head for nits is critical for avoiding an infestation, particularly when other children in your child's school or day care are infected. Make sure your child's school has a policy of notifying parents about lice outbreaks in the school.

Hepatitis A. An inflammation of the liver caused by a virus. This form of hepatitis is spread through food, water, and feces, especially in highly unsanitary conditions. It can also be spread through poor hygiene. A vaccine is available, yet 99 percent of people with hepatitis A recover without treatment.

Hepatitis B. A serious viral infection that causes inflammation of the liver that can lead to scarring of the liver, called fibrosis, or more advanced scarring, called cirrhosis. It is spread or acquired through exposure to infected blood or body fluids, including via sex, childbirth, and needle sharing. A vaccine is available. While there is no treatment for acute hepatitis B, interferon alfa-2b and lamivudine are approved for treating chronic (long-term) hepatitis B.

Hepatitis C. A serious viral infection that causes inflammation of the liver that can lead to scarring of the liver, called fibrosis, or more advanced scarring, called cirrhosis. Unrelated to the other types of hepatitis, hepatitis C is in the Flaviviridae family of viruses. It is transmitted through blood and blood products and less commonly transmitted through urine or sweat. No vaccine or cure is available

HIV. An infection present in the blood and genital secretions of individuals infected with this virus that causes AIDS. HIV is transmitted through needle sharing and when bodily secretions of infected individuals come in contact with tissues, such as those lining the vagina and anal area, or through oral sex. Infected mothers can also spread the disease to their infants during pregnancy or through breastfeeding. No vaccine or cure is available, although antiviral medications may delay the onset of AIDS and decrease the severity of the disease.

Impetigo. A skin infection commonly caused by *Staphylococcus* bacteria and occasionally caused by *Streptococcus* bacteria. The infection causes red, itchy skin with tiny, yellow-fluid-filled sores that crust over when broken. No vaccine exists.

Infectious diarrhea. Gastroenteritis or inflammation of the stomach and intestines caused by a virus, bacteria, or parasite, that can result in severe vomiting and diarrhea. No vaccine exists.

Influenza (flu). A common viral infection that affects the respiratory tract and results in sneezing, congestion, fever, cough, body aches, and overall fatigue. An annual vaccine is available but is not recommended for healthy children.

Listeriosis. A serious illness that threatens pregnant women, the elderly, young children, and those with chronic illness. It is caused by a bacterium, *Listeria monocytogenes*, found in soil and water and is ingested through foods such as raw vegetables, soft cold cuts and cheeses, and uncooked meats. Listeriosis causes a high fever, muscle aches, and sometimes gastrointestinal upset. It can also result in miscarriages and even death in susceptible people. If caught early, it is treated with antibiotics.

Measles. A viral infection that causes cold symptoms, fever, and a red, itchy rash that starts on the face and spreads over the entire body. A vaccine is available as part of the standard vaccination panel for children (it's the first "M" in MMR). With the success of immunization programs, measles are nearly eradicated worldwide.

Mumps. Usually a benign illness that causes swelling of the salivary glands in the cheeks, fever, and sore throat. Mumps is more serious for adolescents and pregnant women. A vaccine is available as part of the standard vaccination panel for children (it's the second "M" in MMR).

Pertussis (whooping cough). This respiratory tract infection is transmitted like a cold and causes months of chronic coughing. A vaccine is available as part of the standard vaccination panel for children (it's the "P" in DPT), and vaccination of adults is under consideration.

Pinworms. A common childhood infection caused by a small, white intestinal worm, *Enterobius vermicularis*. Pinworms cause itching around the anus, disturbed sleep, and overall discomfort. No vaccine exists, but treatments can be given to kill the worms.

Pneumonia. A respiratory infection caused by a bacteria, virus, or fungus that causes congestion and inflammation in the lungs. Pneumonia can be transmitted through tiny droplets in the air, like those that come from a cough or sneeze from someone else, but most cases of pneumonia are caused by aspiration of organisms in our own respiratory tract.

Polio (poliomyelitis). An acute and devastating viral infection that targets the central nervous system, the spinal cord, and the brain and

How Some Germs Are Spread

Contact (with infected person's skin, eyes, nose, or mouth)	**Inhalation** (passing from the lungs, throat, or nose of one person through the air)	**Ingestion** (touching feces or objects contaminated with feces, then touching the mouth)	**Other** (including sex, mother-to-child transmission during birth, and injection)
Chickenpox	Bacterial meningitis	Campylobacter	Gonorrhea
Conjunctivitis	Chickenpox	E. Coli O157:H7	HIV
Impetigo	Cold	Enterovirus	Hepatitis B
Ringworm	Fifth disease	Hand-foot-mouth disease	Hepatitis C
Scabies	Hand-foot-mouth disease	Hepatitis A	Human papillomavirus
	Impetigo	Infectious diarrhea	Syphilis
	Influenza	Pinworms	
	Measles	Polio	
	Mumps	Salmonella	
	Pertussis	Shigella	
	Pneumonia		
	Rubella		

Adapted from *What to Do to Stop Disease in Child Day Care Centers*. Copyright January 1997 by the Centers for Disease Control and Prevention, Atlanta.

can result in weakness or paralysis of the muscle groups. A vaccine is available as part of the standard vaccination panel for children.

Ringworm. A fungal infection on the skin's surface (not caused by a worm). No vaccine exists, but it can be treated with antifungal agents.

Rubella (German measles). An infection that starts with an itchy facial rash. Rubella is serious for pregnant women and can cause miscarriage and birth defects. A vaccine is available as part of the standard vaccination panel for children (it's the "R" in MMR).

Salmonella. A group of bacteria that cause gastroenteritis, food poisoning, and enteric fever, as well as typhoid fever. Some vaccines exist for typhoid, and some infections are treated with antibiotics.

Scabies. An itch "mite" called *Sarcoptes scabiei* that can infect the skin, resulting in uncontrollable itching and discomfort. Scabies is most commonly transmitted through sexual contact, although some physical contact (a hug) may be enough to catch this mite. No vaccine exists, and a prescription cream is necessary to kill the mite.

Tetanus. A bacterium that enters a deep wound and releases a toxin that causes serious paralysis, shutting down the central nervous system. A vaccine is available as part of the standard vaccination panel for children (it's the "T" in DPT), and after completion of the panel, booster shots are required every 10 years to sustain immunity.

Four Steps Parents Can Take to Keep Kids Healthy

Step #1: Immunize your child.

A vital step all parents can take to keep their children well is to get the recommended immunizations when the child is well. Childhood immunizations offer excellent protection against diseases such as diphtheria, pertussis, tetanus, polio, measles, mumps, rubella, *Haemophilus influenzae* type b, chickenpox, and hepatitis B. These vaccines contain an inactivated (killed) agent or a weakened live organism, and they help children to develop antibodies for protection against specific infections.

Understandably, many parents are worried about the risks that are feared to accompany vaccinations, including lingering fear of the hypothetical risk posed by the mercury that was used to preserve some childhood vaccines (a practice that is in the final stages of being phased out). Ever since inoculations were first developed, vaccines have indeed come with risks, including the risk of developing the disease when given live virus or other serious side effects. Most vaccine side effects are mild, and severe ones are very rare, and the use of vaccines has essentially eradicated a number of major childhood diseases that kill. As a risk analyst

Before Vaccines . . .

- Polio paralyzed 10,000 children
- Rubella (German measles) caused birth defects and mental retardation in as many as 20,000 newborns
- Measles infected about 4 million children, killing 3,000
- Diphtheria was one of the most common causes of death in school-aged children
- A bacterium called *Haemophilus influenzae* type b (Hib) caused meningitis in 15,000 children, leaving many with permanent brain damage
- Pertussis (whooping cough) killed 8,000 children, most of whom were under the age of 1

and parent, I believe that the health benefits conveyed by vaccination far outweigh the risks. When parents fail to vaccinate their children, the risk of serious—even deadly—disease epidemics extends beyond them and their families to their neighborhoods and communities. Failure to vaccinate lays the foundation for new epidemics that could result in serious harm to your child. For instance, a decline in vaccination rates in some European countries has led to fatal outbreaks of measles, as reported in *Epidemiology and Infection*.

Step #2: Choose a healthy childcare center.

This is a proactive step that parents can take to reduce a child's risk of bacterial and viral illness. I look for a loving, caring, and clean environment with a nice outdoor play space. While most states focus on health with childcare licensing requirements, I realize that these are *the minimum standards*.

Parents must be aware of all that goes on at the center to ensure the child's health and safety. Let the following questions help guide you as you make the crucial decisions of deciding whether and where to send your kid to childcare.

Is it clean? Do a careful inspection of each center you visit to make sure the workers follow all the rules of cleanliness. Studies document the health benefits of infection control measures in day care—ask whether these are being used. Check in the bathrooms, the kitchen where snacks are prepared or served, the nap area, the workrooms for teachers, and the classrooms. Are paper towels used instead of communal cloth towels? Is liquid soap used instead of bar soap? Does the center look and smell clean? Are there food crumbs on the floor or counters? Is the garbage put away so children cannot access it? Are animals allowed in the school? Make sure that you observe the place when it's full of children so that you get a better sense of what it is like on an average day.

Is hand washing a high priority? Hand washing is the key to stopping the spread of harmful bacteria. Watch to make sure that workers wash frequently as they work with children, serve snacks, come in from the playground, and take children to the restrooms. This one hygiene habit is a good indication of the staff's level of cleanliness.

Is current documentation kept on each child in the center? The

Is Your Child Too Sick for Day Care?

Condition	Guidelines for Time Away from Childcare
Conjunctivitis/Pink eye	24–48 hours after treatment begins
Diarrhea	As child has a watery stool that cannot be contained by diaper, if child can't get to the toilet, if stool contains blood or mucus, or if child also has a fever
Head lice	Until morning after treatment begins; check head daily for next week
Impetigo	24 hours after treatment begins
Mouth sores	Only if child can't control saliva
Rash	If child has fever or until a doctor determines that it is not contagious
Ringworm	Until treatment begins
Strep throat	24 hours after treatment begins and child has no fever for 24 hours
Vomiting	If child has vomited more than twice in 24 hours or is in danger of dehydration

Adapted from *Health & Safety in Childcare: A Guide for Providers in Massachusetts.* Copyright 1995 by the Massachusetts Department of Public Health.

center should have a personal file that includes each child's medical history, immunization records, medications taken and/or treatments needed, allergies, dietary restrictions, and contact information for the child's physician. The center should require that all children be fully immunized.

Does the center encourage or require parents to keep sick children home? This is an important policy because germs are easily spread in close quarters such as childcare centers. When any child comes to the center with a viral or bacterial infection, every child is at risk for catching the same illness. Ask whether the center has a separate area where an ill child can wait to be picked up. The policy of allowing a sick child at school if he is taking antibiotics is not a good one because it promotes both the exposure of well children to sick children and the unnecessary use of antibiotics for viral infections.

Step #3: Manage your child's environment.

There are many things you can do at home to make sure your child's living space is clean and safe, depending on his age and health status and your preferences for home cleaning products. Studies, like one published in 2000, show alcohol and bleach to be very effective disinfectants. Since some people prefer to use natural alternatives, I've included recommendations from herbalist Laurel Vukovic, whose "Home Remedies" column has appeared in *Natural Health* magazine for more than a decade. Laurel suggests using cleaning formulas containing essential oils (extracted from plants), many of which have natural antimicrobial properties.

Toys. If your child is at the age where most plastic toys end up in his mouth, clean them in the dishwasher or with water and a mild hand or dish soap every day or so, and certainly immediately after a toy has been in the mouth of a pet or another child. Periodically use a dishwashing liquid (once a week and immediately after an ill child contacts the toys), and be sure to thoroughly rinse and dry the toys before returning them to your child. Try the following Natural Dish Liquid:

Natural Dish Liquid

- **8 ounces unscented liquid dishwashing soap**
- **2 tablespoons distilled white vinegar**
- **20 drops lavender (*Lavandula angustifolia*) essential oil**
- **20 drops lime (*Citrus aurantifolia*) essential oil**

Combine the ingredients in a plastic bottle and shake well.

Alternatively, run your child's plastic toys through a cycle in the dishwasher to disinfect them, or make a powerful solution of ¼ cup bleach per 1 gallon water and soak plastic toys for at least 3 to 4 minutes. Rinse them thoroughly in clean water, and allow them to air-dry. Bleach does not leave an aftertaste or residue, so don't worry about your child ingesting this from the surface of a toy, as long as it's been thoroughly rinsed and dried.

Changing tables. Once a week, use either your preferred commercial cleaner or the following recipe on your baby's changing table; the essential oils have antimicrobial action and leave a fresh, clean scent.

Changing Table Cleaner

- **2 tablespoons baking soda**
- **2 tablespoons borax**
- **1 gallon hot water**
- **1 teaspoon liquid dishwashing soap**
- **10 drops lavender (*Lavandula angustifolia*) essential oil**
- **5 drops sweet orange (*Citrus sinensis*) essential oil**

Dissolve the baking soda and borax in the hot water. Add the soap and essential oils and use with a sponge to wipe down the changing table. Rinse with clean water.

If your child is ill, wipe the changing table daily with alcohol or ¼ cup bleach in 1 gallon water, rinse with clean water, and allow to air-dry.

Potty seats. Your toddler's potty seat has the potential of being a bacterial breeding ground. Keep germs in check by wiping down the seat with toilet paper after each use and rinsing the bowl thoroughly in hot water before replacing it. Once weekly, or whenever the seat becomes soiled, use either your preferred commercial cleaner or the following cleaner to keep germs at bay:

Potty Seat Cleaner

- **¼ cup baking soda**
- **¼ cup borax**
- **2 tablespoons distilled white vinegar**
- **1 teaspoon liquid dishwashing soap**
- **2 drops patchouli (*Pogostemon cablin*) essential oil**
- **3 drops sweet orange (*Citrus sinensis*) essential oil**

Mix ingredients together and use the cleaner to scrub the potty seat with a sponge. Rinse thoroughly with clean water.

When your child is ill with a bacterial or viral infection, scrub down all parts of the potty seat daily with alcohol or a solution of ¼ cup bleach in 1 gallon water; rinse with clean water and allow to air-dry.

Diaper pails. Diaper pails are obvious havens for bacteria, as soiled diapers sit in them until they are laundered or thrown out. They should be kept away from your child's play area. Remember to wash your hands immediately after changing your baby and disposing of diapers, and wash your baby's hands if he touches his diaper area. To keep odors at bay, use the following deodorizer regularly:

Diaper Pail Freshener

¼ cup borax
¼ cup baking soda
5 drops sweet orange (*Citrus sinensis*) essential oil
2 drops patchouli (*Pogostemon cablin*) essential oil

Mix ingredients together and sprinkle in the bottom of the diaper pail to absorb odors. Store the remainder in a tightly sealed container out of your child's reach.

Once weekly, sanitize your baby's diaper pail using either your preferred commercial cleaner or the following formula:

Diaper Pail Cleaner

1 gallon hot water
¼ cup borax
¼ cup distilled white vinegar
1 tablespoon liquid dishwashing soap
5 drops sweet orange (*Citrus sinensis*) essential oil
2 drops patchouli (*Pogostemon cablin*) essential oil

Mix ingredients together and use to scrub diaper pail. Rinse thoroughly with clean water.

Following the infection, scrub out the diaper pail with alcohol or ¼ cup bleach in 1 gallon water; rinse with clean water, and allow to air-dry.

Children's laundry. Here's a pleasant-smelling mild detergent that will help to reduce germs in your child's laundry:

Mild Laundry Detergent

5 drops lavender (*Lavandula angustifolia*) essential oil
5 drops sweet orange (*Citrus sinensis*) essential oil
½ cup baking soda
½ cup borax
½ cup powdered castile soap

Add the essential oils by the drop to the baking soda and mix with a metal spoon. Put mixture through a hand sifter to thoroughly distribute the oils. Add the borax and powdered soap and again sift well. Store in an airtight container. Add ½ cup to a full load of laundry.

When laundering items that are soiled with urine or feces, add ½ cup bleach and use hot water.

High chairs. Because high chairs often trap crumbs of food and remain damp following spills, they require extra attention. After each meal, wipe down the high chair with a sponge and hot water, carefully removing any food debris. Follow up with either your preferred commercial cleaner or the following solution:

All-Purpose Spray Cleaner

1 teaspoon borax
1 teaspoon baking soda
1 cup hot water
2 tablespoons distilled white vinegar
½ teaspoon liquid dishwashing soap
¼ teaspoon lavender (*Lavandula angustifolia*) essential oil
¼ teaspoon sweet orange (*Citrus sinensis*) essential oil

Dissolve the borax and baking soda in hot water and cool to room temperature. Pour into spray bottle, add the remaining ingredients, and shake well. Spray liberally onto the high chair and wipe off with a clean, damp sponge. This solution can also be used to clean walls and other surfaces.

Step #4: Teach proper hand washing.

Studies have shown that the simple act of hand washing throughout the day can prevent the spread of disease to a significant degree. Show younger children how to wash between each finger with plenty of mild

> **When Illness Strikes**
>
> - If family members aren't well, make sure they have separate towels, eating utensils, dishes, and drinking glasses for the duration of their illnesses. Wash these items thoroughly before anyone else uses them.
> - Wash all bed linens and clothing of sick family members separately.
> - If possible, open the child's bedroom windows to ventilate the room while she recuperates.
> - Disinfect any items that have been handled by the sick child. Soak thermometers in alcohol, and clean toilet seats, potty chairs, and high chairs with alcohol or a bleach solution.
> - Stock up on tissues when family members get colds, and place wastebaskets nearby for discarded tissues.
> - Remind family members to cover their noses and mouths when they cough or sneeze and to wash their hands afterward. Some child-care centers teach children to cough into the crook of the arm so germs are not transferred onto the hands. This is a great technique to use at home with little ones.

liquid soap and warm water, and teach them to use nail brushes to reach under fingernails where hidden bacteria may lurk. Suggest they count to 20, say their ABCs, or sing a favorite song—anything that will occupy them while they engage in this proven method of disease prevention. Provide a stack of toss-away paper towels in the bathroom for family members to use for drying. This is just one more preventive step toward keeping "bad" bacteria from spreading among family members.

As you teach your family members the importance of hand washing, go over the following healthy hygiene rules:

- Each member of the family should wash their hands before eating.
- Before preparing food or feeding children, adults should wash their hands. After handling raw meat, adults should wash their hands with an antimicrobial soap (either a commercial product or a natural one—but one that will kill the germs; see chapter 5 for more about handling raw meat).
- All members of the family should wash their hands after using the bathroom or changing a baby's diapers. All diapers, baby wipes, tissues, and dirty or soiled laundry should be stored or disposed of in a sanitary manner, and garbage cans and diaper pails should be kept out of the reach of curious toddlers.
- If you have any contact with bodily secretions (including nasal mucus, phlegm, vomit, diarrhea, or blood), wash your hands immediately.
- Remind adults who come into your home to wash their hands before any contact with babies or small children.

Using Your Child's Risk Quotient

Now that you have a better understanding of what you and your child are up against with germs and resulting illnesses, I have identified a variety of common illnesses that are bacteria-related or treated (or mistreated) with antibiotics. I give a brief description of each illness, explain what causes it, and describe the signs and symptoms. I also let you know when to call your doctor and whether an antibiotic is the best possible treatment. As with the illnesses for adults (discussed in chapter 3), Chris D. Meletis, N.D., a naturopathic physician who serves as dean of naturopathic medicine and chief medical officer at the National College of Naturopathic Medicine in Portland, Oregon, has outlined some excellent preventive measures and self-care remedies that you can use at home, depending on your child's level of risk.

As you consider these strategies, remember to always check with your child's pediatrician *before* your child tries any herbs or supplements, and take into account any particular factors that may be especially important for your child, such as allergies for which there may be possible reactions to new things. Similarly, if your child has a chronic health condition, be particularly careful with herbs and supplements. You must also be exceptionally cautious about reading and following the instructions on any labels for children every time; if the instructions say to take with food or after eating, then do. Don't give children under 4 lozenges or cough drops, and monitor any child using lozenges for the first few times to ensure that he does not choke on them. See "About the Remedies in This Chapter," opposite, for more cautions and tips to consider.

Risk Quotients 1 through 4

If your child is basically healthy and scored in RQs 1 through 4 in the Personal Health Risk Profile and does not have a chronic condition that requires ongoing medical care, then the proactive strategies, alternative therapies, and natural remedies suggested below may help to prevent or

About the Remedies in This Chapter

Don't give a product to your child unless you have specific instructions from a reliable source like your child's pediatrician. Before giving your child any herbal or conventional product, always read the labels. Here are some other things to consider:

Acidophilus (*Lactobacillus acidophilus*). If your child has any serious gastrointestinal problems that require medical attention, check with your pediatrician before supplementing. If you child is taking antibiotics, they should be taken at least 2 hours before supplementing.

Aspirin and NSAIDs. Aspirin and ibuprofen (Children's Advil and Children's Motrin) should always be given with food to avoid stomach upset. Because of the link to Reye's syndrome, a life-threatening illness that may lead to brain and liver damage, children and teenagers with fever or flu should be given only Tylenol, never aspirin or NSAIDs. (See "Watch Out for Reye's Syndrome" on page 213.) If your child has aspirin sensitivity or asthma, do not give ibuprofen, as it may cause wheezing.

Echinacea (*Echinacea purpurea* or *E. angustifolia*). Do not give to a child who is allergic to closely related plants such as ragweed, asters, and chrysanthemums. Since echinacea stimulates the immune system, do not give to a child with tuberculosis or an autoimmune condition such as lupus or multiple sclerosis.

Licorice cough drops. Do not give to children with high blood pressure, diabetes, and some other chronic conditions. Do not give cough drops to children under 4.

Magnesium. Do not give to children with renal disease.

Vitamin C (ascorbic acid). Do not give to children prone to kidney stones.

Vitamin E. Be sure to use top-quality vitamin E, either the d-alpha or mixed tocopherol types (not synthetic d,l-alpha vitamin E).

Zinc lozenges. Give after eating to avoid nausea. Do not give lozenges to children under 4.

end an acute illness such as a sore throat, ear ache, bronchitis, or diarrhea. Just as we discussed in chapter 3, find your child's Risk Quotient under each condition and consider the other steps prior to that RQ as well. It's important to always be ready to use conventional medical therapies for serious illness and feel comfortable about calling your child's pediatrician. If you are not interested in trying natural or alternative therapies, then the self-care suggestions may still be helpful in preventing illness.

Risk Quotient 5

If your child has a compromised immune system; a chronic illness such as diabetes, asthma, renal disease, hepatitis, or AIDS (but not limited to these; ask your child's pediatrician about others); or an RQ of 5, work with your child's pediatrician to help your child stay well. The conventional medical doctor is someone you must trust to run the necessary tests, make an accurate diagnosis, and give your child the best medical treatment—particularly antibiotics when they are necessary—to end infections early on.

Now find the optimal approach for your child's individual situation and decide which health problems should send you to the doctor immediately and which are safe to self-treat and monitor with the simple strategies listed. Even if these common illnesses are not currently impacting your child, following the basic prevention strategies that I explain may still improve your child's health and that of your family.

Bites and Stings

What Is It? The bites of some insects contain venom that can trigger an allergic response, while others carry disease that can be bacterial, viral, or parasitic.

What Causes It? When the insect bites and injects venom or other foreign agent into your child's skin, this triggers an allergic (immune) reaction. In all cases, the area should be cleaned with rubbing alcohol with care so the stinger is not pushed into the skin even further, but do not delay the removal of any stinger if rubbing alcohol is not readily available. In the case of bees, stingers should be scraped off with a blade or fingernail but not removed with tweezers, which may squeeze more venom out of the venom sac. In contrast, always remove ticks using tweezers because this increases the chance of removing the tick's mouthparts, which, if left in the skin, can cause persistent irritation. Also be very careful to avoid rupturing the ticks, and wear gloves if you can while removing ticks to avoid contamination with tick fluids that may be infected.

Signs and Symptoms: Following an insect bite or sting, your child may experience itching or mild swelling. A more serious reaction includes continued and uncontrolled itching, burning, continued swelling (of the earlobes, lips, and throat, among others), and difficulty breathing. Sometimes a bite or sting can lead to hives (raised welts), nausea, fever, painful joints, and swollen glands.

Prevention and Treatment:

RQ 1 **Observe the child.** Once you've removed the stinger and cleaned the affected area with alcohol, put ice on the wound to reduce swelling, and keep a watchful eye on your child for signs and symptoms of an allergic reaction. Call your doctor immediately if any symptoms arise. If your child has difficulty breathing, call 911 for emergency care.

Prevent emergencies. If there's a family history of severe allergies to bee stings, ask your doctor about keeping an allergy kit (EpiPen) containing epinephrine at home and at school in case of a severe reaction.

Epinephrine is a synthetic form of adrenaline used for treating anaphylactic shock caused by severe allergic reactions. The EpiPen contains an injectable form of epinephrine that is easy to use and can help your child live a normal life.

RQ 2 **Make a baking soda paste to ease itching.** Mix baking soda and water to make a thick paste, then spread this on the bite. Use as needed to help ease itching and inflammation.

RQ 3 **Use an antihistamine cream.** Rub an antihistamine cream or gel, such as one containing diphenhydramine (Benadryl), on the bite to reduce swelling and alleviate subsequent itching without the diphenhydramine systemically entering the blood stream. This cream is available over-the-counter at most grocery and drug stores.

Take an antihistamine. If your child is prone to allergies from bites or stings, give him diphenhydramine (Benadryl), an antihistamine that will reduce the allergic response.

Repel the bugs—safely. A variety of commercial insect repellants contain DEET (N,N-diethyl-m-toluamide), a chemical insect repellant that has been proven effective; the American Academy of Pediatrics recommends using preparations containing 10 percent or less DEET on

A Word about Ticks

If you find a deer tick on your child, remove it using tweezers by firmly grasping the tick and carefully pulling the entire tick off the skin. Do not use your fingers to remove a tick. Put the tick in a jar of rubbing alcohol in case your doctor needs to test it for Lyme disease. Observe your child for any unusual signs or symptoms, such as a round, red rash (erythema migrans) that looks like a bull's-eye. Erythema migrans is often accompanied by fever, headache, stiff neck, body aches, and fatigue.

children. Alternatives include Avon's Skin-So-Soft, which studies show is less effective but many people swear repels mosquitoes. Soybean oil, available at natural foods stores, may also repel mosquitoes when rubbed onto the skin. Researchers from Iowa State University presented findings at the 222nd national meeting of the American Chemical Society that catnip oil may be even more effective at preventing some types of mosquito bites than DEET. Whatever product you use, avoid applying it on children's faces and hands so they won't inhale or ingest the repellant.

RQ 4 **Ward off bugs.** Citronella (*Cymbopogon nardus*), a lemon-scented plant from Asia, is used in many items to ward off insects. You can buy citronella candles at most grocery and hardware stores. Use these anytime your child is playing outdoors to help keep bugs away. Some people find that fresh basil (*Ocimum basilicum*) from the garden can keep bugs away. Take several leaves and rub these on your child's clothes as a natural insect repellent.

When to Call the Doctor: Call your doctor or 911 if your child shows any signs of a severe allergic reaction: difficulty breathing; swelling of the earlobes, lips, or throat; confusion; rapid heart rate; or nausea or vomiting.

Bronchitis (Acute)

What Is It? Acute bronchitis is a common childhood illness caused by inflammation and irritation of the bronchial tubes that results in chest congestion, mucus production, difficulty breathing, and coughing.

What Causes It? Contrary to what most parents believe, acute bronchitis is often not a bacterial infection that is remedied by a prescription from your pediatrician. It's usually a virus that causes acute bronchitis, although it can sometimes be caused by chemical irritants in the air (cigarette smoke, smog, industrial chemicals), allergens (allergy triggers including dust, dust mites, feather pillows, mold, mildew, and animal dander), and infections. *Mycoplasma* and *Chlamydia*, two of the infectious organisms that cause acute bronchitis, are being studied for their roles as possible causes of asthma.

Signs and Symptoms: Your child may have a cough with production of mucus, which can be thick and yellow. He may have a fever and fatigue, along with wheezing and shortness of breath. If the bronchitis is severe, it can progress into pneumonia, which is inflammation of the lungs due to viruses or bacterial infection. Pneumonia demands a doctor's medical treatment.

Prevention and Treatment:

RQ 1 **Increase rest.** When your child has acute bronchitis, the first action you should take is to put her to bed. The increased rest for a day or two will allow your child's body to recover more quickly from the impact of symptoms.

Force fluids. Make sure your child stays well-hydrated with fluids such as chipped ice, water, clear liquids, juices, broth soups, gelatin, Pedialyte, and ice pops. The additional liquids are necessary to help thin mucus so your child can expel the secretions. Stagnant mucus in your child's bronchial tubes is more likely to get infected.

RQ 2 **Use a humidifier.** Keep a hot steam humidifier running in your child's room to increase moisture in the air and help to loosen sticky secretions. Be sure to keep the humidifier clean and dry

Viral or Bacterial?

With viral bronchitis, your child may run a low-grade fever or no fever at all. There is little mucus coming from the lungs at the onset of the illness, and your child may not feel very sick. With bacterial bronchitis, however, your child will feel very ill and have a higher fever (over 101° F) and a deep cough. The mucus will be very dark, usually green or brown, and comes from the lungs, not from the back of the throat. You should see your doctor for proper diagnosis and treatment.

between uses to prevent the growth of bacteria, fungi, and molds. And make sure bedding and carpeting don't get wet, as mold and bacteria can form there, too.

Try an expectorant. Guaifenesin, an over-the-counter ingredient found in many popular cough syrups such as Robitussin, is an excellent expectorant. This medication helps to thin mucus so the child can expel it easily.

RQ 3

Try a decaffeinated herbal tea. Some people find that a tea brewed from garlic (*Allium sativum*) and ginger (*Zingiber officinale*) loosens phlegm and can be safely used long-term. Simmer 2 cloves of garlic and 2 to 3 slices of ginger root in 1 cup of hot water for 15 minutes. Add pasteurized honey and lemon to flavor and serve warm with meals to prevent upset stomach.

Rub the congested chest. Blend 3 to 4 drops of either common thyme (*Thymus vulgaris*) or eucalyptus (*Eucalyptus globulus*) essential oil in 1 tablespoon sesame oil or other food-grade oil. Gently rub the oil on your child's chest to reduce congestion; cover with a warm cloth that you've placed in the drier for a few minutes. If you do not have essential oils, if your child is sensitive to them, or if you prefer, try the over-the-counter remedy Vicks VapoRub on the chest only.

RQ 4 **Sip mullein tea.** Mullein (*Verbascum thapsus*) is an amazing herb that is soothing to the mucous membranes and helps to thin and bring up the sticky mucus. Mullein is filled with mucilage, a naturally occurring chemical that lines the mucous membranes of the respiratory tract, protecting against irritation and inflammation. It also contains small amounts of tannins, which improve resistance to infection, and saponins, which are natural expectorants.

Boost immunity. Acute bronchitis may follow an upper respiratory tract infection such as a cold or the flu. If your child is ill with either of these conditions, help her to resist further infection. Give your child a variety of fresh fruits and vegetables, which are rich in healing antioxidants, and make sure she gets regular exercise and play, adequate sleep, and less stress.

Give your child foods high in magnesium. Magnesium is one mineral that's important for a number of biochemical reactions related to lung function. Some studies, like one in the *Journal of Asthma*, have found that a low intake of magnesium in the diet may result in asthma and chronic obstructive airway disease. Magnesium may have a powerful influence over lung function with several antiasthmatic actions, such as relaxing smooth muscles in the airway, dilating bronchioles, and reducing airway inflammation. Foods high in magnesium include almonds, avocadoes, black-eyed peas, cashews, kidney beans, lima beans, oatmeal, pecans, shredded wheat, soy flour, soybeans, tofu, and walnuts.

When to Call the Doctor: If your child has difficulty breathing, shortness of breath, a fever higher than 101° F, or is coughing up green or blood-stained mucus, call the doctor. Also check with the doctor if your child has a continuous cough or wheezing. These symptoms may indicate asthma, a condition that affects more than five million children. Any child with a history of asthma, wheezing, or cystic fibrosis should be under a doctor's care if she is also suffering from bronchitis.

Colds

What Is It? Colds are the most common illness among children. This respiratory virus lasts around 1 week, and children, especially preschoolers, may have between five and eight infections annually. They are also one of the most common childhood illnesses that send children and their parents to the pediatrician for antibiotics in the hope of quick relief. Colds are particularly prevalent among children attending childcare.

What Causes It? No matter what your child's symptoms—green mucus, fever, or croupy cough—almost all colds are caused by one of more than 200 different virus strains. These viruses may also affect your

Is It a Cold or Sinusitis?

When your child's congested nose and cough continue after 7 to 10 days, you may want to see if it's sinusitis. Sinusitis is an inflammation of the nasal sinuses, those hollow cavities within the cheekbones, around the eyes, in the forehead, and behind the nose. While their main job is to warm, moisten, and filter the air we breathe, when there is inadequate drainage of the sinus cavities, mucus stagnates and can become infected. Symptoms include headache, congestion, thick discolored mucus, fatigue, and fever.

If your child has sinusitis, your doctor can help you establish a treatment plan that may include decongestants, expectorants, nasal steroid sprays, and antibiotics, if necessary.

child's airway, sinuses, throat, voice box, and bronchial tubes and can even cause nausea and vomiting at the early stages of the cold. Parents often mistake these for symptoms of a bacterial infection.

Signs and Symptoms: A cold usually begins abruptly with great discomfort in the throat followed by such symptoms as clear, watery nasal discharge, sneezing, a tired sensation (malaise), and sometimes fever. Postnasal drip causes the sore throat and cough that accompany colds.

Colds are usually self-limiting, which means that they go away on their own. But fatigue, stress, or the virus itself may promote a bacterial infection, which can weaken the body's immune system and require treatment with an antibiotic. Increased rest, reduced stress, and staying well-hydrated, however, can help to prevent bacterial infections from developing.

Sometimes your child may have allergic rhinitis (hay fever) or a sinus infection, which can mimic a cold. If the symptoms begin quickly and are over within about 7 days, then it is usually a cold, not allergies. If your child's cold symptoms last longer than a week, check with your pediatrician to see if he may have developed an allergy or sinus infection.

Prevention and Treatment:

RQ 1 **Increase rest.** Help your child get to bed earlier and take naps throughout the day when a cold first begins. It is during the deepest stages of sleep that the body is revitalized and tissue damage is repaired. In fact, lack of sleep is associated with reduced immune function.

Boost liquids. Your child needs plenty of liquids to help thin the thick mucus, making it easier to expel. Encourage water, clear liquids, ice chips, ice pops, gelatin, juices, and broths. Avoid bananas, citrus, peanuts, and dairy foods, which may increase mucus production; also avoid any known food allergens.

RQ 2 **Try saline nose drops.** To help relieve nasal congestion, try saline nasal drops. These drops can be purchased over-the-counter and are effective, safe, and nonirritating, even for children. To use, instill several drops into one nostril, then immediately bulb-suction that nostril. Repeat the process in the other nostril.

Consider supplements. Supplements that have been shown to decrease the duration of colds include vitamin C, echinacea (*Echinacea purpurea* or *E. angustifolia*), elderberry (*Sambucus nigra*), and zinc lozenges (especially zinc-gluconate with glycine).

Soothe the throat. Give your child warm decaffeinated tea with lemon and pasteurized honey to help soothe his irritated throat.

RQ 3 **Use a hot steam vaporizer.** Use a hot steam vaporizer (not a cool mist) in the bedroom at night. This warm, humid environment will help to keep your child's nose and chest clear, making it easier to breathe. Be sure to clean the humidifier daily to prevent the growth of bacteria, fungi, and molds.

Try healing aromatherapy. Blend 3 to 4 drops of either common thyme (*Thymus vulgaris*) or eucalyptus (*Eucalyptus globulus*) essential oil in 1 tablespoon sesame oil or other food-grade oil. Gently rub the oil on your child's chest to reduce congestion; cover with a warm cloth that you've placed in the drier for a few minutes. Or gently rub Vicks VapoRub on your child's chest and cover with a warmed cloth; do not apply to your child's nose. Menthol, the key ingredient, can help to open stuffed breathing passages.

Prop his head while sleeping. Let your child sleep on two pillows to help mucus drain from the back of the throat instead of "choking" him.

RQ 4 **Practice prevention.** While adults come down with only one or two colds a year, children typically have five to eight colds because of their underdeveloped immune systems. But an immature immune system isn't the only thing that makes kids vulnerable. They also tend to spend lots of time with other children and aren't always careful about washing their hands, which makes it easy for colds to spread. Consider using alcohol-based hand sanitizers like Purell to keep germs under control. Remember, also, to keep kitchen and bathroom countertops clean, especially when someone in your family has a cold (see chapter 5 for details), and discard used tissues right away.

When to Call the Doctor: If your child's symptoms last longer than a few days or if he has a chronic illness, such as asthma or diabetes, that can place him at a higher risk for complications, call your doctor. Usually, children get sicker than adults with colds and suffer more from complications such as asthma and bronchial and ear infections. Call your doctor immediately if your child appears lethargic, excessively fatigued or despondent, has a fever higher than 101° F, a fever that lasts more than 3 days, vomiting or abdominal pain, unusual sleepiness, severe headache, neck pain, difficulty breathing, ear or throat pain, a purplish, spotty rash, or feels that light bothers his eyes.

Conjunctivitis

What Is It? Conjunctivitis is a very common eye complaint, especially in children. It happens when the conjunctiva, a transparent membrane that lines the inside of the eyelid and covers the whites of the eye, becomes inflamed.

What Causes It? Conjunctivitis can be caused by allergies, dry eyes, irritation, a virus, or a bacterial infection known as "pinkeye." Pinkeye is common in childcare centers or crowded classrooms, but both viral and bacterial conjunctivitis are contagious, caught from exposure to someone with this disease. No matter what the cause, call the doctor for an evaluation and accurate diagnosis. You do not want to second-guess anything to do with your child's vision.

Signs and Symptoms: With conjunctivitis, your child will have redness, tearing, a "gritty" feeling when blinking, itching, burning, and swelling of the eye and eyelid. With bacterial conjunctivitis, there is usually a thick, yellow-green, mucuslike discharge that crusts over the eye and glues the eyelid together. Viral conjunctivitis usually affects both eyes, while bacterial pinkeye may only affect one. Allergic conjunctivitis leaves the eyes red, itchy, and watery, but there is no thick yellow-green discharge.

Prevention and Treatment:

RQ 1 **Keep the eye clean.** Use a clean, moist tissue to wipe the discharge away from the irritated eye. Dispose of the tissue immediately, and wash your hands to avoid spreading the infection.

Isolate your child. Children with conjunctivitis should not use the same bar soap, hand towels, or bath towels as others in the household. If your child has bacterial conjunctivitis and your doctor prescribes antibiotics, your child still may be contagious for 2 days after treatment begins. Keep him home from childcare or school for a few days or until your doctor feels he is no longer contagious, and use any antibiotics prescribed as directed. Make sure to wash your hands frequently, or you may be the next victim of pinkeye.

Use over-the-counter eye drops. If your doctor believes that an allergy is causing the conjunctivitis, ask about whether your child might benefit from taking oral antihistamines or from medicated eye drops to ease the itching and inflammation. If your doctor confirms that a virus is causing the problem or does not suspect allergies, ask about saline eye drops such as Visine Tears, Tears Naturale, or Artificial Tears to ease the discomfort. Many over-the-counter eye drops contain a decongestant that will remove the redness and make your child's eyes feel better, but they will make it more difficult for the doctor to diagnose the underlying cause of redness. See your child's pediatrician about any eye redness your child experiences before using any eye drops containing a decongestant, and ask a pharmacist to help you identify appropriate brands. With all eye drops, never touch the tip of the dropper to the eye, as germs can spread to the product and infect others.

RQ 2 **Use moist heat compresses.** Warm, moist compresses can help to alleviate the inflammation that causes the pain and itching. Apply a compress to the eye every 3 or 4 hours to ease burning and wipe away crusts. If applying to both eyes, use a clean cloth for the second eye. Never reuse the same compress; place immediately into the laundry and wash your hands to avoid spreading the infection.

RQ 3 RQ 4 Work with your child's doctor.

When to Call the Doctor: If you suspect conjunctivitis, contact your child's pediatrician to determine the cause. Inform the doctor whether the infection is associated with blurred vision, heavy eye tearing, thick mucus in the eye, or fever. Only your doctor can determine which type of conjunctivitis your child has, and the treatment is different depending on whether it's viral or bacterial. Rare types of conjunctivitis can lead to blindness if left untreated.

Cuts and Scratches

What Is It? Cuts and scratches are everyday occurrences for most active children. Whether from stubbing a toe, skinning a knee, or bumping into the edge of the coffee table, they all have one commonality—they are physical injuries that result in an opening or break in the skin. Bacteria can enter the wound, causing infection.

What Causes It? There can be many causes of breaks in the skin from a scratch, cut, or puncture to a scrape, splinter, or bump. Anything that puts stress on the skin can weaken it, causing it to tear or break open.

Signs and Symptoms: Your child may have torn skin, or the skin may be scraped off entirely, depending on the type of wound. There may be a lot of blood, particularly if the wound is on the face or head, or no blood at all. Most cuts, scratches, and other wounds are painful for children, but with some wounds, your child may not have a lot of pain even though the wound is more serious. If the wound oozes, has an odor, shows spreading redness, has warmth or swelling pain, or forms a yellow or green scab, it could be infected and should be checked by a doctor.

Prevention and Treatment:

RQ 1 **Give immediate first aid.** When your child is cut, try to cover the wound with a cloth so she does not see the opening, which can make it seem worse. If it is bleeding, cover the wound with a clean cloth and apply pressure; hold for 2 or 3 minutes until the bleeding has subsided. For a deep wound, one that is bleeding profusely or requires a tourniquet, seek medical care immediately. It's important to allow small wounds to bleed for a minute or so to get rid of infectious agents and to keep all wounds—large or small—clean and dry.

Make the assessment. If the wound is gaping open or on the child's face, seek medical attention immediately. If it is not gaping and is small, self-care can probably speed healing. If in doubt, call your doctor, especially when it comes to facial wounds that could result in scarring. If the wound occurred outdoors or as a result of a rusty metal object, or if it is a puncture wound, consult a physician because of the possibility of tetanus. Be sure your child is up-to-date on immunizations, or a booster may be needed.

Clean the wound. Apply an antiseptic spray, such as Bactine, and cover with a gauze bandage. Try not to let the gauze stick to the open wound or it may irritate it.

Elevate the wound. Elevating the wound, in combination with direct pressure, can help to slow bleeding. Elevation also helps prevent swelling, supports the natural healing process, and is particularly important if the cut is on your child's arm, hand, leg, or foot.

RQ 2 **Coat it with aloe.** Aloe gel or the sticky residue from a crushed aloe leaf (*Aloe barbadensis*) may help to resolve pain and speed healing.

RQ 3 **Use vitamin E.** The oil of a vitamin E capsule may help to soothe the skin, minimize scarring, and relieve itching once a scab forms. After 4 days of healing, apply the oil and rub gently over the scab.

RQ 4 **Boost EFAs.** Essential fatty acids (EFAs) are essential to healthy skin and are available in fish and flaxseed oils, which contain omega-3.

When to Call the Doctor: Most wounds heal with regular self-care. But if the wound becomes more painful, inflamed, red, or has pus or a green liquid draining from the opening, call your doctor. You may wish to have the wound cultured to determine whether an antibiotic is necessary.

Diaper Rash

What Is It? While diaper rash is frightening to the new parent, this bright red patch on a baby's bottom is really nothing more than inflamed skin or dermatitis.

What Causes It? Diaper rashes result from babies remaining too long in wet diapers and plastic pants that trap wetness next to their skin. The warm moist area provides the perfect environment for microbes to grow, resulting in two types of diaper rashes. *Irritation rashes* occur when bacteria, normally present in stool and urine, break down to form ammonia, which irritates baby's delicate skin, and *yeast rashes*, which result when yeast (fungi) that are normally found on the skin take over and grow out of control.

Signs and Symptoms: Both types of diaper rash are characterized by reddish, puffy, and perhaps slightly warmer skin in the diaper region. Irritation diaper rashes are pink or red and resemble sunburn; yeast diaper rashes are usually bright red and sometimes extend outside of the diaper area. You may notice that your baby is more uncomfortable than usual, especially during diaper changing. A baby with a diaper rash will usually fuss or cry when the diaper area is washed or touched.

Prevention and Treatment:

RQ 1 **Keep her clean.** Change diapers frequently—especially while your baby has the irritation. Wash her skin gently with water after each changing to remove any waste from the skin. Avoid perfumed soaps, opting instead for a mild, gentle variety; rinse it thoroughly from the skin and dry your baby thoroughly after the bath.

Let the area air-dry. Place baby on a soft quilt or thick towel with the diaper area exposed and let her bottom air-dry—the longer the better.

Avoid known triggers. If your child experiences repeated cases of diaper rash, pay attention to solid foods that have recently been introduced, and try eliminating them to see if the condition improves.

Wash your hands frequently. If yeast is causing the diaper rash, this infection can spread to you and others if you're not vigilant about hand washing.

Use a mild ointment to boost healing. Petroleum jelly, zinc oxide, and vitamins A and D are the time-tested ingredients found in many commercial products to prevent and treat diaper rash; these include Vaseline, Vitamin A & Vitamin D Ointment, and Desitin. These products should be used as directed on clean skin to help keep it in good condition.

Avoid using plastic pants or tight-fitting clothes. When waste is held tightly against baby's body, this can cause increased irritation. Plastic pants hold the wetness in—next to baby's skin—and can worsen diaper rash.

RQ 2 **Try different types of diapers.** You may find that keeping your baby in cloth diapers increases the chances of diaper rash. If you use disposable diapers, try different brands until you find the one that works best with baby's skin. Some disposable diapers absorb urine and hold it away from baby's skin, while others are not as absorbent.

Rinse cloth diapers. Try adding ¾ cup vinegar to the washer's rinse cycle to help remove alkaline irritants. If you use a diaper service, ask them to do the same.

RQ 3 **Avoid powders.** While our grandmothers thought that powders and cornstarch helped to keep baby dry, we now know that these stick to the tiny folds in a baby's skin, forming the perfect breeding ground for bacteria to grow. Powders can also irritate baby's lungs and upper respiratory system.

RQ 4 **Boost flora.** If you are a nursing mother and have taken antibiotics recently, ask your doctor about acidophilus supplements (*Lactobacillus acidophilus*) to replace the normal, good bacteria (flora) that live in our intestines. Normally, the intestinal flora regulates digestion and bowel movements. But yeast also inhabits the intestines. When the environment is healthy, the bacterial flora and yeast keep each other in check. But the good bacteria, along with the bad, get depleted when you take antibiotics, causing the yeast to multiply and results in problems such as yeast infections. You might also try to up your and your child's consumption of yogurt with live cultures to try to help normal flora return more quickly.

When to Call the Doctor: In most cases, you can easily heal your baby's diaper rash within a few days of beginning treatment. But if the rash worsens or does not respond to treatment after 2 or 3 days, call your doctor. If your child has a fever, blisters, or bleeding with the rash, it's best to call your doctor to make sure your baby does not have a secondary infection. Sometimes food allergies can result in diarrhea and diaper rash. Keep a list of any new foods or liquids your baby has had and give this to your doctor to help speed up a diagnosis. Your baby may need to see a dermatologist if the condition persists.

Diarrhea

What Is It? Diarrhea, or loose, watery stools, can make your child very uncomfortable, causing frequent trips to the bathroom and overall weakness or fatigue.

What Causes It? There are different causes of diarrhea. One common cause in young children is infection from viruses such as rotavirus and adenovirus. Direct contact with other children in a crowded childcare facility easily spreads viral diarrhea from one child to the next. Bacteria such as *E. coli*, *Salmonella* (often carried by reptilian pets), and *Campylobacter* can cause diarrhea, as can *Giardia lamblia* and *Cryptosporidium*, two parasites that cause the intestines to work overtime. Contaminated food or water, food allergens, and medications may also cause this common gastrointestinal problem. In most cases, including bacteria-related, antibiotics are not necessary to resolve the illness.

Signs and Symptoms: Your child has diarrhea if he has more frequent bowel movements than normal and the stools are loose or watery. He may experience abdominal pain or cramps, fever, headache, or nausea and vomiting.

Prevention and Treatment:

RQ 1 **Stay hydrated.** Encourage your child to drink plenty of liquids, including ice chips, water, ice pops, clear broths, gelatin, juices, and electrolyte replacement drinks like Pedialyte. One easy way to tell if your child is becoming dehydrated from a lengthy spell of diarrhea is to weigh him daily before you dress him. Report to your doctor immediately if you notice a rapid decline in weight or if your child is urinating less frequently than normal.

Keep hands washed. You can help prevent the spread of viral diarrhea by washing your hands and encouraging your child to wash his hands. Because viral diarrhea spreads easily, it's a good idea to keep your child home from school or day care if he has diarrhea.

RQ 2 **Use the B.R.A.T. diet.** Give your child bland foods including bananas, rice or rice cereal, applesauce, and dry toast. As he is able to keep these foods down without discomfort, add other food from his regular diet. Avoid spicy foods and dairy products for several days after the diarrhea has ended.

RQ 3 **Add yogurt.** Yogurt can add good bacteria (flora) back into the intestinal tract after a bout of diarrhea. Check products for a label that includes the words "active live cultures." (But wait until the diarrhea has resolved before adding any dairy products.)

RQ 4 **Add good bacteria.** Ask your doctor if your child might need to take acidophilus (*Lactobacillus acidophilus*) or *Bifidobacterium bifidum* capsules or powder to replenish his body with good bacteria. Lactic acid bacteria are often called *probiotics* and serve to maintain the health of the intestinal tract by producing acids and other compounds that inhibit the growth of disease-causing bacteria.

When to Call the Doctor: Diarrhea can be a serious condition. If your child's symptoms persist or worsen within 24 hours, call your doctor. If symptoms include lethargy or dehydration, or if your child does not urinate normally, has a rapid heart rate, has blood or mucus in the stools, has a persistent or high fever (higher than 101° F), experiences persistent abdominal pain, or if the diarrhea is accompanied by vomiting, contact your pediatrician immediately.

Ear Infections

What Is It? Ear infections, the common name for acute otitis media (AOM), account for 35 percent of all pediatric visits, and pediatricians generally see one patient suffering from ear pain every day.

What Causes It? Viruses may cause up to 80 percent of ear infections, and antibiotics have no effect on these. For the bacterial-related infections, the culprit is *Streptococcus pneumoniae*, which results in 7 million cases of ear infection each year in the United States. Thirty percent of these bacteria are now resistant to drugs in the penicillin family, and resistance to other medications is growing. Ear infections can occur first with a viral infection, after which a secondary bacterial infection may occur.

Signs and Symptoms: With an ear infection, your child may have ear pain, difficulty sleeping, irritability, clear or yellow-green mucus in the nose, low-grade fever (lower than 101° F), or ear drainage. The most painful part of an ear infection is at the very beginning. This is because the sensory nerve endings in the eardrum respond to increased pressure with pain, and after the eardrum stretches a little, the pain will not be so intense. If you notice your child tugging a lot on his ear, it's probably worthwhile to have it checked.

Prevention and Treatment:

RQ 1 **Use a hot water bottle to ease pain.** While your child is lying on his side, place a cloth on his sore ear, then gently lay a hot water bottle on top of the cloth. Test the hot water bottle first to make sure it radiates warmth but is not too hot. The warmth will help to soothe the pain and reduce inflammation.

Numb the pain. Ibuprofen, a nonsteroidal anti-inflammatory drug

Watch Out for Reye's Syndrome

While Reye's syndrome is rare (1 case per one million children), it is something all parents should know about. Reye's is usually preceded by a viral infection such as bronchitis, throat infection, diarrhea, or chickenpox. Symptoms include nausea, vomiting, lethargy, delirium, and rapid breathing. As the illness progresses, the child's breathing becomes sluggish, and the child becomes comatose with dilated pupils. At the first sign of any of these symptoms following a viral infection, call your doctor for immediate treatment.

(NSAID) found in Children's Motrin and Children's Advil, and acetaminophen, found in Children's Tylenol, Tempra, and Panadol, are useful in treating symptomatic ear pain. Because inflammation contributes to the discomfort of ear infection, ibuprofen is often recommended for its anti-inflammatory effects. Ibuprofen can be especially helpful at nighttime because its duration of action is 6 to 8 hours, whereas the duration of acetaminophen is only 4 hours.

RQ 2 **Try over-the-counter medications.** Some doctors believe that guaifenesin, an expectorant found in over-the-counter cough medications such as Robitussin, helps to relieve blockage of the eustachian tubes; ask your pediatrician.

RQ 3 **Boost liquids.** Encourage your child to drink more liquids to help thin mucus.

RQ 4 **Chew on it.** If your child experiences frequent ear infections, consider a chewing gum containing xylitol, a natural sugar that appears to prevent bacterial growth and attachment. For prevention, give one stick per day; during treatment, give two to three sticks per day.

When to Call the Doctor: If your child has a fever higher than 101° F, appears lethargic, excessively fatigued or despondent, complains of neck or head pain, or has a discharge coming from the ears, contact your pediatrician for treatment. With a cold, the nasal passages swell, and your child may have subsequent ear pain. But with a bacterial ear infection, the germs go up through the eustachian tube and into the middle ear space. Once the germs land in the thick mucus, they start to breed, causing pus to form, which fills the middle ear space and results in inflammation and pain. The doctor will probably practice watchful waiting and, if necessary, prescribe an antibiotic for treatment of an ear infection. If the eardrum is perforated, your pediatrician may prescribe antibiotic drops with prednisone (a steroid used to reduce inflammation). Any time an eardrum is perforated, you must take extreme caution to prevent anything, including water, from entering your child's ear while it is healing.

Flu

What Is It? The flu is a viral infection that attacks your child's respiratory system—her nose, throat, bronchial tubes, and lungs. This infection can cause severe complications, particularly pneumonia.

What Causes It? Three different types of viruses—influenza A, B, and C—are responsible for the flu. Type A causes the deadly influenza epidemics that appear every few decades. Type B is responsible for smaller, more localized outbreaks. Type C is the least common and causes only mild symptoms. Your child can become infected when someone with the flu coughs or sneezes or if your child touches something the person has handled.

Signs and Symptoms: Your child may sneeze, cough, ache, and have a high fever and chills. It may seem like a cold with the nasal congestion and difficulty breathing, only greatly intensified. A low-grade fever is common with the flu and may last almost a week.

Prevention and Treatment:

RQ 1 **Put your child to bed.** The first few days of the flu are no fun, and bed is the best place for your child. Increased rest will allow her body to recover more quickly from the impact of symptoms.

Stay hydrated. Force fluids during the flu, including chipped ice, water, clear liquids, juices, broth soups, gelatin, Pedialyte, and ice pops. Liquids help to thin mucus and replenish the body's fluids lost by fever so your child does not get dehydrated.

Numb the pain. Give your child an analgesic such as acetaminophen (Children's Tylenol, Tempra, or Panadol) or ibuprofen (Children's Advil or Children's Motrin) to reduce pain and fever. Ibuprofen may work best as it reduces fever, relieves pain, and fights inflammation.

RQ 2 **Ease congested breathing.** Guaifenesin is the main ingredient in over-the-counter cough remedies such as Robitussin and works to keep mucus thin so it can flow freely in your child's congested nasal passages and bronchial tubes. This may help her breathe easier so the discomfort is reduced.

RQ 3 **Consider supplements.** Chewable vitamin C tablets with bioflavanoids or rose hips (which are the most easily absorbed forms) and zinc lozenges (especially zinc-gluconate with glycine) can help to support your child's immune function.

Try echinacea or elderberry. *Echinacea purpurea* or *E. angustifolia* and *Sambucus nigra* may help to ease your child's symptoms and shorten the duration of the flu.

Use a decongestant. If your child is really congested, ask your pediatrician if you can give her a decongestant, which may help to shrink the nasal passages and reduce congestion. Common ingredients of over-the-counter decongestants include phenylephrine and pseudoephedrine.

Use saline drops or nasal sprays. Saline drops or nose sprays can help to clear out thick mucus in the nasal passages, helping your child breathe easier. When mucus stagnates in the nose and sinus cavity, it acts as a breeding ground for bacteria to grow, resulting in an infection.

When to Call the Doctor: Usually a child will get well without further medical treatment if you ensure plenty of rest and liquids. For high-risk children, the flu can be life threatening. Call your pediatrician if your child starts showing symptoms of the flu and has any of the following conditions:

- Asthma or other lung conditions
- Cardiovascular disease
- Diabetes or chronic kidney disease

Your doctor may recommend the flu shot for a high-risk child over the age of 6 months. If your child isn't at risk but is around someone who has a chronic illness or compromised immune system, adults in the house (who aren't allergic to eggs) should consider getting flu vaccinations to keep the infection from spreading in your home.

If your child is having difficulty breathing, has a productive cough with dark mucus, or has a high fever, call your pediatrician. Bacterial pneumonia is sometimes mistaken for the flu, and antibiotic therapy is necessary for recovery.

Impetigo

What Is It? Impetigo is a common childhood bacterial infection of the skin that can occur just about anywhere on the body. Highly contagious, it is usually found around the child's buttocks, arms, mouth, or nose.

What Causes It? Blame the bacteria *Streptococcus* (strep) or *Staphylococcus* (staph) for most causes of mild impetigo. When your child's skin is irritated from scratching, allergic rhinitis, the excessive drooling with teething, or the open sores of a diaper rash, the bacteria congregates in that moist place and begins to multiply.

Signs and Symptoms: You may notice small red spots that look like tiny pimples on your child's skin. These spots may become itchy and quickly turn into blisters that burst open, leaking a sticky, honey colored secretion. Sometimes a yellow crust can form on top of the impetigo. These circular spots can grow as large as a quarter.

Prevention and Treatment:

RQ 1 **Keep it clean.** Using a tissue or cotton ball, wash the infected area of skin several times each day with an antibacterial soap and warm water. Cover the impetigo sores with gauze bandage after cleaning. For sores on the face or in the nose, make sure they are thoroughly cleaned several times a day; cover with gauze if possible. Throw the tissue, cotton ball, and old bandages away after cleaning and wash your hands thoroughly.

Talk about cleanliness. If your child can keep his hands off the infection, the chances of it spreading to other family members or friends are minimal. Encourage your child to wash his hands frequently, and make sure fingernails are clipped so they can stay clean.

Try a topical antibiotic. Sometimes your doctor will have to prescribe a topical antibiotic. Bactroban is one prescription antibacterial cream that's commonly used and may resolve most mild cases of impetigo.

RQ 2 **Keep skin healthy.** It's important to know that bacteria do not usually penetrate unbroken skin. You can help to prevent skin irritation by cleaning all wounds with soap and water. Keep open wounds covered, and use a mild antibacterial ointment like Neosporin if desired.

RQ 3 **Prevent infections.** Wash your child's sheets, clothes, and towels separately in hot water during the infection to prevent other family members from catching the impetigo.

RQ 4 Work with your child's doctor.

When to Call the Doctor: If the impetigo is spreading to different parts of your child's body or if it is worsening after 3 days of treatment, with increased itching and oozing secretions, check with your pediatrician to see if antibiotics are needed. Because impetigo can spread to others, keep your child away from other children for at least 3 days and until the infection begins to clear.

Sinusitis

What Is It? Sinusitis is an inflammation of the nasal sinuses, those hollow cavities within the cheekbones, around the eyes, in the forehead, and behind the nose.

What Causes It? The sinuses' main job is to warm, moisten, and filter the air we breathe. When there is inadequate drainage of the sinus cavities, mucus stagnates and can become infected. When the action of the mucus coat is altered by trauma, drying, irritating chemicals, or any other factor, the nose, sinuses, and lower respiratory tract become more susceptible to infection.

When your child has a cold or viral infection, the nasal mucous membranes become compromised and sinusitis can develop. Other irritants include air pollution, smoke, airborne allergies, dry or cold air, and ozone.

Signs and Symptoms: With sinusitis, your child may have headache, increased pressure around the eyes, cheeks, and forehead, along with cold symptoms, green or yellow mucus, pain in the upper molars, cough, and a fever of 101° F or even higher.

Prevention and Treatment:

RQ 1

Increase rest. Bed rest may help your child recover from sinusitis faster. Encourage early bedtime and naps during the day to allow your child's body a chance to heal from the infection. Also let your child sleep on two pillows so the sinus drainage does not pool in her throat.

Avoid irritants. Keep your child and her bedroom clean (including nightly showers), and avoid exposure to any known irritants to relieve the symptoms of sinusitis.

Boost liquids. Your child will experience thicker mucus with sinusitis. Drinking clear liquids, such as water, diluted juices, Pedialyte, and broths will help to thin the mucus, making it easier to dispel. Watch out for iced drinks, as some people find that cold or iced drinks can aggravate the condition. Ask your pediatrician about whether any specific foods should be avoided.

RQ 2 **Use an over-the-counter expectorant.** Try over-the-counter cough medicines that contain the expectorant guaifenesin, which helps to thin mucus associated with nasal congestion and drainage. Be sure to get medication that contains only guaifenesin, such as Robitussin, unless your doctor has prescribed otherwise. Some cough medications contain drying agents that may worsen the sinus problem.

Try saline nose drops. To help relieve sinus congestion, use saline nasal drops. These drops can be purchased over-the-counter and are effective, safe, and nonirritating, even for children. To use them, instill several drops into one nostril, then immediately bulb-suction that nostril. Repeat the process in the other nostril. You can also ask your pediatrician about the Proetz method of irrigating your child's sinuses to help alleviate nasal congestion and stuffy nose.

Soothe the throat. Give your child warm decaffeinated tea with lemon and pasteurized honey to help soothe the irritated throat associated with sinusitis. Licorice cough drops, available at most grocery stores and pharmacies, help to soothe swollen throats and also thin mucus.

RQ 3 **Use moist heat.** Apply warm compresses to your child's forehead and sinus area to help alleviate the pain and pressure, but be careful that they are not too hot.

Try healing aromatherapy. Blend 3 to 4 drops of either common thyme (*Thymus vulgaris*) or eucalyptus (*Eucalyptus globulus*) essential oil in 1 tablespoon sesame oil or other food-grade oil. Gently rub the oil on your child's chest to reduce congestion; cover with a warm cloth that you've placed in the dryer for a few minutes. If you do not have essential oils or if your child is sensitive to them, try the over-the-counter remedy Vicks VapoRub on the chest only.

Consider supplements. Vitamin C, echinacea (*Echinacea purpurea* or *angustifolia*), and zinc lozenges (especially zinc-gluconate with glycine) can help to bolster the immune system.

RQ 4 **Use a decongestant.** Decongestants can provide much relief, especially if your child's sinus passages are swollen and congested. The decongestant can shrink blood vessels, reduce swelling in the nasal passage, and open the mucous membranes in the nose. Your child will feel less pressure in the sinuses and head and breathe more clearly.

Opt for EFAs. Essential fatty acids (EFAs) are not manufactured by the body but are essential to sinus health because they reduce swelling (and pain) associated with the allergic response. They work by aiding in the production of prostaglandins that counter inflammation. EFAs are available in fish and flaxseed oils, which contain omega-3.

When to Call the Doctor: If your child's symptoms last longer than 1 week, if she is running a fever higher than 101° F, or if she is having trouble breathing, call your pediatrician. Sometimes sinusitis can trigger bronchitis and even asthma, resulting in coughing and wheezing. You should expect that the pediatrician may prescribe an antibiotic and that radiology tests may be needed if the case is complicated.

Sore Throat

What Is It? Sore throat is one of the most common medical complaints, sending millions of children to the doctor's office each year for diagnosis and treatment. Sore throat can make it hard to swallow, difficult to breathe, and even make eating a chore.

What Causes It? Your child's nose and throat are constantly defending against outside elements and bacteria. Most sore throats are caused by irritated mucosa in the throat. In some cases, when bacteria settle in the nose, they are seized and dragged off to battle stations called lymph glands where the good white cells are kept. More good blood comes to the area. There, the concentration of good white cells can overwhelm the bacteria. But when the lymph material swells, this causes the symptom your child feels—a painful

Mononucleosis

One cause of sore throat is mononucleosis (mono), which is an acute viral infection typically caused by the Epstein-Barr virus (EBV) or less frequently by Cytomegalovirus (CMV) and results in a high temperature, sore throat, and swollen lymph glands. Mono is spread by saliva, thus the label of "the kissing disease," and commonly occurs during the teenage years (from age 15 to 17), although anyone can be affected.

With mono, your child may initially feel lethargic, run a low-grade fever, and have a sore throat. As the disease progresses, the throat pain worsens, and the tonsils may swell and have a whitish-yellow, pus-like coating on them. Sometimes a light pink rash occurs with mono.

During the physical examination, your doctor will feel an enlarged spleen or liver that is also tender to the touch. A blood test will show unusual appearing white blood cells, which will help to confirm the diagnosis of mononucleosis. Sometimes the liver enzymes are abnormal with this condition, too.

Unless there is a secondary infection, there is no treatment for mono other than rest, sometimes for as long as a month. Treat the symptoms with the remedies listed in the "Colds" and "Flu" sections (pages 199 and 214, respectively), and relieve pain with over-the-counter analgesics (except aspirin). The illness usually resolves within 4 to 6 weeks without medication.

throat. (Strep throat is a more serious cause of sore throat. See page 226.)

Either a virus or bacteria can cause a sore throat. The most important difference between viral and bacterial causes is that bacteria respond well to antibiotic treatment, but viruses do not. Some of the most common causes of sore throat include sinus drainage, postnasal drip, a "dry" throat from taking an antihistamine, tonsillitis (discussed on page 230), a swollen uvula (the flap of skin in the back of the throat)—usually scratched by foods such as crackers, chips, or bagels—infectious mononucleosis or "mono" (see "Mononucleosis," opposite), and strep or streptococcus group A. Gastroesophageal reflux disease (GERD) is another cause of sore throat. This happens with regurgitation of stomach acids into the back of the throat and is particularly a problem when your child lies down at night. If you suspect GERD, take your child to his pediatrician.

Signs and Symptoms: Your child may complain about a scratchy or sore throat or may not say anything and just refuse to eat or drink. He may be fatigued, achy, feverish, and have a runny nose. The glands in the neck may be enlarged, and he may have a headache.

Prevention and Treatment:

RQ 1 **Avoid irritants.** Air pollution, weather changes, smoke, dust mites, and even animal dander can all cause inflammation and swelling of the throat and nose. If your child has allergies or sinusitis, make sure all known triggers are removed from his bedroom to avoid worsening the problem.

Make your child comfortable. For most types of sore throat, time will heal it if your child gets increased rest. Boost liquids such as water, chipped ice, juices, clear broths, gelatin, and ice pops. Warm decaffeinated tea with pasteurized honey may help to coat the throat and soothe it.

Numb the pain. Give your child an analgesic, such as ibuprofen (Children's Advil or Children's Motrin) or acetaminophen (Children's Tylenol), to ease the pain and tenderness.

RQ 2 **Use a hot-mist humidifier.** When the throat is swollen and dry, breathing or even swallowing become difficult. The added moisture from a hot-mist humidifier can help your child sleep sounder and breathe easier while he recuperates from the infection. Be sure to clean the humidifier daily to avoid a buildup of bacteria, fungi, and molds.

Soothe the throat. Look for throat lozenges that have clear instructions for children. Lozenges containing benzocaine are available over-the-counter. This ingredient helps to numb the sore throat pain and may help your child to eat and drink more during the illness.

RQ 3 **Try zinc lozenges.** Zinc is a key nutrient necessary to fight infection. Medications or poor diet may cause a deficiency of zinc. Whole foods high in zinc include seafood, eggs, meats, whole grains, wheat germ, and seeds. While the studies are not conclusive, some people find that zinc lozenges (especially zinc-gluconate with glycine) help to soothe painful sore throats and may even reduce symptoms because of an antiviral effect in the mouth and nose.

RQ 4 **Take an allergy medication.** Sometimes a constantly sore throat is the result of postnasal drip (mucus) that stagnates in the back of the throat during sleep. Ask your doctor whether a decongestant or antihistamine (or combination medication) may help resolve this problem.

Ask about GERD. New studies are pointing to gastroesophageal reflux disease (GERD) as a cause of chronic sinusitis with symptoms of thick mucus in the throat, hoarseness, and difficulty swallowing. GERD may also result in a chronic, scratchy or sore throat upon awakening.

GERD usually occurs at night when your child is lying down. Normally, a valve between the esophagus and the gastric system prevents stomach acids from backing up into the esophagus. In GERD, this valve does not work properly. The stomach acids reflux, or back up, into the esophagus, causing irritation and inflammation. Symptoms of GERD include excess mucus production, trouble breathing, a scratchy sore throat, heartburn, and wheezing. Your doctor can run tests to diagnose GERD, and treatment, which may include foods to avoid, can help to resolve the problem.

When to Call the Doctor: The most serious type of throat infection is epiglottitis, which is caused by a bacterium that targets part of the voice box (the larynx), resulting in inflammation or swelling that actually closes the airway. Never put anything like a tongue depressor in your child's mouth if he is complaining of difficulty swallowing, even if he may not be able to verbalize the complaint and the only symptom is drooling or a change in his voice. Putting in a tongue depressor may trigger a spasm, which can close off the upper airway. If your child has difficulty swallowing or speaking and labored breathing, seek emergency medical attention. Call your pediatrician if your child's throat continues to hurt after 2 days, or if your child is running a fever either higher than 101° F or for longer than 3 days, has swollen tonsils, enlarged lymph glands, a severe headache, difficulty breathing, or vomiting. Another serious condition is strep throat (see page 226). While symptoms vary, you should contact your pediatrician if your child has difficulty swallowing, has extremely tender lymph nodes, or white patches in the back of his throat.

Strep Throat

What Is It? Strep throat (or "strep") is a common bacterial throat infection, especially with elementary-age children (ages 6–12). It is extremely contagious.

What Causes It? You can blame the *Streptococcus pyogenes* bacteria for causing strep throat. These bacteria spread through airborne droplets when your child is sitting in class when another child with the infection coughs or sneezes. Your child could get infected when he touches a doorknob then wipes his nose or puts gum into his mouth.

Signs and Symptoms: Your child may start with a sore, scratchy throat that often flares into a very painful throat upon swallowing. Other common symptoms include low-grade fever (lower than 101° F), aches, swollen lymph glands, swollen and coated tonsils, and occasionally abdominal pain. Sometimes your child can have strep throat without any symptoms at all. But if left untreated, strep may lead to serious problems such as abscess in the tonsils, scarlet fever, which must be treated with antibiotics to avoid incurable rheumatic fever that can damage heart valves and lead to other chronic problems including kidney damage. If you're in any doubt, immediately consult your doctor, who can perform throat cultures to determine whether the sore throat is caused by strep.

Prevention and Treatment:

RQ 1 **Increase rest.** If your child has strep throat, make sure he gets more rest than normal. Sleep helps the body fight infection and heal faster.

Boost liquids. Make sure your child drinks lots of water, juices,

The Strep Test

The symptoms of strep throat are very similar to tonsillitis and other viral throat infections. Ask your doctor about the rapid test kit that checks throat secretions for bacterial infections in the office within minutes. If your child tests positive for strep bacteria, antibiotic treatment can be started right away. If the rapid test is negative, your doctor may still want to do a throat culture and send it to a laboratory for analysis. Cultures have to grow, so you will wait from 1 to 2 days to hear the final results. Make sure any medicine is completely finished because stopping antibiotics early can create strains of resistant bacteria and make future episodes more difficult to treat.

Pedialyte, and clear broths. Chipped ice and ice pops give your child extra fluids and also help to numb the throat pain.

Use paper products. To avoid infecting other family members or reinfecting the child once he's well, the infected child should use paper cups and towels and throw them away immediately after use. Keep a stash in the bathroom and kitchen.

RQ 2 **Moisturize the air.** Strep throat can make it difficult to swallow or breathe. Added moisture to the air with a cool-mist humidifier helps to keep the inflamed and irritated mucous membranes in the throat from drying out, which would cause even more irritation and pain. Clean the humidifier daily to keep bacteria, fungi, and molds from growing.

RQ 3 **Use warm salt water rinses.** Older children can rinse the back of their throats with warm salt water (½ teaspoon salt to 8 ounces warm water). Instruct your child to carefully swish the water in the back of the throat but not to gargle. Gargling may injure the uvula, which can be very swollen and sensitive. Be sure to remind him to spit the water out after rinsing his throat.

RQ 4 **Boost immune function.** Make sure your child is eating a variety of nutritious foods, particularly fresh fruits and vegetables high in the antioxidant vitamins A, C, and E. Consider supplementing with zinc lozenges (especially zinc-gluconate with glycine) and with echinacea (*Echinacea purpurea* or *E. angustifolia*) and vitamin C, which boost immune function. See "Dietary Reference Intakes" on page 164.

When to Call the Doctor: When your child has symptoms of strep throat, call your doctor, particularly if the sore throat lasts more than 2 days. Strep throat needs immediate attention and antibiotic therapy. After your child has finished the antibiotics, if there are still symptoms, check with your pediatrician. In rare cases, another course of medication is necessary to fully kill the strep bacteria.

Sty

What Is It? When your child awakens with a red, painful bump on the eyelid, your child might have a sty. In most cases, a sty is a relatively benign, common condition that will resolve itself with home care. If you're not sure whether it is a sty, call your pediatrician.

What Causes It? Sties are infections near the root of the eyelash caused by bacteria. Your child may have more than one sty at a time or several in succession. (Not all lumps on the eyelid are sties; they could be another type of swelling called a chalazion, which is caused by blockage of a small gland that produces part of the tear layer.) To be certain, have your child's pediatrician diagnose the condition.

Signs and Symptoms: A sty usually starts small then quickly fills with pus, causing it to swell and making it difficult to see clearly. It may cause tearing in the eye, along with pain from the inflamed tissue.

Prevention and Treatment:

RQ 1 **Use moist heat.** Put moist heat compresses on the sty to alleviate the pain and swelling, but make sure that they are not too hot. When the sty comes to a head and bursts on its own, clean the eye area with a damp cotton ball. If pus is draining into the eye, immediately flush it with saline or water to prevent the bacteria from infecting the eye and see your pediatrician. If pus is not draining into the eye, then avoid flushing or rubbing the eye to keep from spreading the bacteria.

RQ 2 **Try saline drops.** Ask your pediatrician about using over-the-counter eye drops such as Artificial Tears, Tears Naturale, or Visine Tears to keep the irritated eye moist; these drops can be used several times a day during the course of the sty.

RQ 3 **Wash hands.** Although sties are not thought to be contagious, make sure your child washes his hands frequently throughout the day and uses paper towels. Also remind him to keep his hands out of his eyes—and off his face in general to avoid irritating the delicate tissue.

RQ 4 **Boost immunity with healing nutrition.** Make sure your child's diet includes a variety of fresh, colorful fruits and vegetables, whole grains, and legumes that are high in phytochemicals, which are natural food components that have health-boosting properties.

Consider supplementing. Talk to your doctor about supplementing with vitamin C, echinacea (*Echinacea purpurea* or *E. angustifolia*), and zinc lozenges (especially zinc-gluconate with glycine), to boost your child's immune function. See "Dietary Reference Intakes" on page 164.

When to Call the Doctor: If the sty worsens, interferes with your child's vision, or will not burst on its own, call the doctor. Your child may need to have a doctor lance the sty to drain the pus and to relieve the pain and pressure. If the sty returns or if your child has multiple sties, your doctor may prescribe antibiotics.

Tonsillitis

What Is It? When some of us were very young, removing the tonsils was commonplace, especially for those children who had suffered with a few painful tonsil infections. Today, doctors know that tonsils are a normal part of the body's immune system, helping to filter out harmful bacteria, viruses, or other particles that can cause infections.

The tonsils are made of lymphoid tissue and are part of the immune system. Located on each side of the throat, the tonsils act as filters, guarding the entrance to the lower respiratory system. Sometimes, though, they become clogged, swollen, and infected.

Tonsillitis is especially prevalent among children from ages 3 to 6, as their immune systems are getting established. Others at high risk for this common infection include children in crowded childcare centers and those prone to respiratory tract infections.

What Causes It? Sometimes a low-grade infection stimulates the immune system to form antibodies against future infections. But when your child's tonsils are overwhelmed by a bacterial or viral infection, they swell and become inflamed. Most cases of tonsillitis are caused by the bacterium *Streptococcus pyogenes*. A host of other respiratory viruses—such as the Epstein-Barr virus (EBV), which causes mononucleosis—can also cause tonsillitis.

Signs and Symptoms: Your child's tonsils will become swollen and red, and he may have a severe sore throat and difficulty swallowing. Other symptoms include headache, fever, chills, body aches, swollen neck glands, and fatigue. You may notice patches of white discharge or even blood on your child's infected tonsils.

Prevention and Treatment:

RQ 1 **Make your child comfortable.** While there is no treatment for the virus that causes some forms of tonsillitis, you can make your child comfortable by increasing rest, ensuring that he drinks plenty of liquids, and using analgesics, such as acetaminophen (Children's Tylenol), to ease the throat pain.

Numb the pain. Sucking on chips of ice may help to relieve some of the discomfort from tonsillitis, as may ice cream, sherbet, or flavored ice pops. Avoid hot liquids, as they may irritate the throat.

RQ 2 **Keep the air moist.** If your child has nasal congestion and postnasal drip with the tonsillitis, using a hot-mist humidifier in his bedroom may help. But remember to clean and dry the humidifier daily, as bacteria, fungi, and molds can flourish.

RQ 3 **Try nasal irrigation.** If sinus drainage or postnasal drip is causing tonsils to become inflamed, nasal irrigation with saline solution (salt water) may help bring relief. In a study published in *Clinical Pediatrics* on children age 5 and older who had sinusitis, postnasal drip, or nasal blockage, nasal irrigation with a saline solution was helpful.

RQ 4 **Use lozenges.** Look for children's throat lozenges, available over-the-counter, that contain benzocaine (unless your child is allergic to it). This ingredient helps to numb the pain of tonsillitis and may help your child to eat and drink more comfortably.

Boost immune function with nutrients. Make sure your child's diet is filled with a variety of fresh fruits, vegetables, dairy products, and protein. If your child is a picky eater, talk to your doctor about vitamin and mineral supplements.

Get more rest. When children do not get enough sleep, their resistance toward disease can lessen, and they become an easy target for any virus or bacterial infection. Put bedtime earlier for a few weeks so your child catches up on lost sleep.

When to Call the Doctor: Call the doctor immediately if there's any suggestion of difficulty swallowing or breathing because tonsils can enlarge to the point that the airway can become obstructed. If your child has tonsillitis resulting from a viral infection, the only thing you can do is treat the symptoms, make your child comfortable, and wait for the virus to run its course. If the tonsillitis is from a strep infection, antibiotics are necessary. Antibiotics typically need to be taken for 5 days or longer, and stopping antibiotics early can fail to kill the bacterial culprits, allowing the infection to come back and causing potentially serious complications. Surgery, while not generally recommended, is used in more serious situations, such as if your child's breathing is hindered.

Tooth Decay

What Is It? Tooth decay is a bacterial disease; it eats away at your child's teeth and results in cavities. Children are especially vulnerable to tooth decay if they eat between meals, take a bedtime bottle of milk or juice, or have poor dental hygiene. Left untreated, tooth decay can destroy the internal structures of your child's tooth, resulting in tooth loss.

What Causes It? When your child drinks sweetened drinks or eats sugary foods, the sugars stay on the teeth and gums, feeding the bacteria that cause plaque. When plaque is not removed, it mineralizes and turns into tartar. Together, plaque and tartar cause more damage, irritating the gums and resulting in gingivitis. If gingivitis continues over a period of time, tooth decay results.

"Baby bottle" tooth decay gets its name from the fact that babies who go to sleep with a bottle in their mouths are more prone to this problem. It is caused by the frequent and long-term exposure of a child's teeth to liquids containing sugars. While the baby sleeps, the flow of saliva decreases. This causes sugary liquids to congregate around the baby's teeth for a long period of time, feeding the plaque-causing bacteria.

Signs and Symptoms: With tooth decay, you may see tiny holes or discolorations in your child's teeth. With baby bottle tooth decay, it is usually the front teeth that are initially affected. If left untreated, your child may complain about a tooth hurting when she eats hot, cold, or sweet foods.

Prevention and Treatment:

RQ 1 **Teach your child good dental hygiene.** Even before your newborn has visible teeth, pediatric dentists recommend that parents clean the baby's mouth after each feeding, or at least twice a day (morning and evening). Take a clean damp cloth or 2-inch square piece of gauze and wrap it around your index finger. Moisten the cloth with water and gently wipe the gum pads in your baby's mouth. This will help to reduce food debris and the oral bacteria that form in the mouth. Never leave a bottle in your child's mouth once she falls asleep.

As soon as your child has her first tooth, you need to set up a regular tooth-brushing routine. This should be after each feeding or snack (or at least twice a day), using an extra soft brush and fluoride toothpaste. By age 3, or when your child can handle holding a fork or pencil, let her brush her own teeth for a few minutes before you finish the job.

You should start flossing your child's teeth daily (every night) by age 2 and continue doing this until the child becomes good enough at flossing to take over the job, usually around age 6 or 7. At that time, the dentist or hygienist can teach the child how to use floss correctly, and you should reinforce this at home.

Do not share toothbrushes or tubes of toothpaste, store toothbrushes in separate locations to avoid spreading illness, and replace your child's toothbrush after the illness has passed.

RQ 2 **Watch snacks.** Most children eat several small meals a day instead of three larger meals. But all-day snacking keeps the child's mouth acidic and promotes tooth decay. If your child cannot brush after every snack, choose the following foods that are at low-risk for causing cavities: raw vegetables (broccoli, carrots, cauliflower, celery), cheeses (Swiss, Monterey Jack, cheddar, cream, and cottage), peanuts or natural peanut butter (no sugar added), popcorn, nuts and seeds, hard-boiled eggs, plain yogurt without sugar (you can mix in fresh fruit), fresh fruits, and natural fruit juices (no added sugar). If your child's gums bleed during brushing, talk to your dentist about brushing and increase intake of vitamin C-rich foods and dark green vegetables.

RQ 3 **Ask about sealants.** Always use a fluoride toothpaste, and when your child is around age 6, ask your dentist about the need for sealants. These dental products are effective in protecting pits and fissures without harming the tooth enamel. Taken early on, these preventive measures can dramatically reduce cavities and dental problems in later life.

RQ 4 **Boost your child's intake of calcium.** Make sure your child gets plenty of the following calcium-rich foods that help to keep teeth strong: dairy products (milk, cheeses, yogurt, and ice cream), greens (mustard, kale, and turnip), okra, oranges, salmon (canned with bones), sardines (canned with bones), tofu (processed with calcium sulfate) and other soy-based products, and calcium-enriched foods. If your child is a picky eater, ask your pediatrician about a multivitamin-mineral supplement.

When to Call the Dentist: The American Dental Association recommends taking your child to the dentist within 6 months of the eruption of her first tooth—and no later than her first birthday. After that initial visit, the child should routinely see the dentist for preventive cleaning and treatments twice a year. If your child has any signs of tooth decay including pain, sensitivity, or holes in the teeth, make an appointment immediately to get the problem treated. Early treatment of tooth decay can stop the damage and save the tooth.

5

HYGIENE IN THE HOME

I believe that healthy hygiene at home is important for keeping you and your family well. But let's face facts: Life is sometimes extremely hurried and harried! Who has time to clean every nook and cranny in her home every day? As a busy professional and parent, I'd rather spend my free time enjoying my family and hobbies than be a slave to housecleaning. That's why I recommend *targeted* hygiene—focusing on the household "hot spots" where dangerous bacteria lurk. If the hot spots are clean, then you can feel safe with housekeeping that suits your personal preferences, whether that's weekly, monthly, or seasonal.

The knowledge that disease-causing germs inhabit your kitchen and bathroom might make you want to reach for antibacterial cleaners to protect yourself and your family. In fact, some Americans are now so obsessed with being clean that a new psychological disorder called *myso-*

phobia has emerged; this is the severe fear of coming into contact with dirt. While most of us don't have mysophobia, we are insecure about germs and believe that cleaner *always* must mean better. In general, that's true—but let's not forget about overkill.

Some scientists are now waving red flags when it comes to antibacterial products, warning that they may be contributing to the resistance crisis. Initially these agents were viewed as miracle substances that destroyed harmful germs without any side effects; some studies show that they may work like antibiotics and may leave behind stronger bacteria that the products can no longer kill.

Originally, antibacterial agents were used in hospitals to help stop the spread of infection; today they are a multimillion-dollar industry. More than 76 percent of liquid soaps on the market now contain antibacterial substances, most frequently triclosan (see page 36). According to data from ACNielsen, Americans purchase $540 million worth of antibacterial soaps, hand cleaners, and detergents each year. In fact, more than 700 antibacterial products are currently on the market, including cut-

A Healthy Home

Some basic safety measures to take around your house include ensuring that the heating, ventilation, and air conditioning systems in your home function properly by cleaning them and changing the filters as recommended. Keeping your home free of pests is also important because they carry germs and allergen-producing substances, including some that may trigger asthma attacks. And make sure that you take care of any spills, moisture problems, or water damage immediately in such places as poorly ventilated basements, around walls with ongoing water leaks, and in other water-damaged areas.

ting boards, kitchen wipes, dishcloths, sponges, kitchen sprays, hand wipes, dishwashing liquids, toilet disinfectants, garbage bags, cling wrap, children's toys, and mattress covers and pillows. Some of these products simply are simply overkill. While we may think they're fighting infection, the net result for you and your family may be a long-term possibility of promoting difficult-to-treat bacterial illness.

Where Harmful Bacteria Hide

While bacteria are microscopic, the problems they can cause can be enormous. Take *E. coli*, for example. These bacteria thrive in the intestinal tracts of certain animals, including humans and cattle, and it was not until 1982 that *E. coli* was first recognized as a cause of human illness. In the past 5 years, studies that document *E. coli* infections have provided a much better understanding of their impact on the population, leading to current estimates by the Centers for Disease Control and Prevention (CDC) that tens of thousands of Americans suffer at least mild symptoms each year from *E. coli* infections.

Fully 80 percent of infectious diseases are transmitted by touch, so it bears repeating that frequent hand washing is your best protection from illness. The simple friction generated by skin rubbing against skin, along with warm water and plain soap followed by thorough rinsing and drying, sloughs the potentially harmful bugs down the drain and out of your way.

It's easy to forget how important hand washing is—but imagine this scenario: Your child uses the bathroom and does not wash her hands carefully. *E. coli* hitches a ride with her into the kitchen and is introduced to everything she touches—the refrigerator handle, the cupboard shelf, and the warm, damp sink where she finally deposits her empty glass.

Unknowingly, you may rinse a piece of fruit for her, resting it on an *E. coli*-laden surface—after all, it looks clean—just long enough to allow the bacteria to jump to their new host: a shiny red apple. After your child takes a few bites, she passes the apple to her best friend to finish. Within 2 or 3 days, her friend wakes up with nausea, vomiting, abdominal cramps, and diarrhea. Was it a bad apple? Another case of stomach flu? Maybe. But the chances are great that these symptoms were caused by the transmission of *E. coli*.

Other bacteria are also present in our environment and, like *E. coli*, can wreak havoc with the human body if they find their way past its natural defense systems. These germs hide in the places you'd least expect them, like the kitchen sponge that is usually damp and contains tiny food particles. Bacteria can live for more than 2 days in a damp sponge because it provides a moist surface that is easy to cling to and has a steady supply of nutrients. Your garbage disposal is another hot spot—a moist place where food particles accumulate—and every time you turn on the disposal, bacteria may be sprayed out of the drain and into the air in the form of tiny aerosol particles (unless you have the disposal covered). The telephone receiver handle and buttons also can harbor a variety of germs. Toilet handles, sink faucets, and bathroom doorknobs are other danger zones.

In an intriguing 1998 study done at the University of Arizona in Tucson, researchers examined 15 homes for more than 7 months to find the most contaminated areas. Ironically, the toilet seat was last on the list of monitored areas. Those with the highest bacteria count included sponges and dishcloths, 7 billion bacteria per average-sized sponge; kitchen faucet handles, 229,000 bacteria per square inch; cutting boards, 62,000 bacteria per square inch.

While these numbers are startling, remember that disease doesn't result from the mere presence of bacteria, even when they occur in staggering numbers. First they have to get on you and in you. Let's take a look, then, at some of the most common household pathogens, where they hide in your home, and what symptoms to watch for to see if they've entered your body. Once you know what you're up against, you can take steps to stay well, no matter what your Risk Quotient. With just a few precautionary measures, you *can* live in harmony with germs.

Common Food-Borne Pathogens

Campylobacter

Where They Hide: In your home, *Campylobacter jejuni* is usually found on surfaces that have come into contact with raw meat, poultry, shellfish, and unpasteurized milk. Common household surfaces include kitchen counters, cutting boards, and dirty dishes used in the preparation of the raw foods.

Signs and Symptoms: Within a few days to 2 weeks after eating infected foods, you may have headaches, fever, and aches or muscle pain, followed by nausea, vomiting, diarrhea, and abdominal pain. *Campylobacter* is the most common bacterial cause of diarrhea in the United States.

Clostridium perfringens

Where They Hide: Small numbers of *Clostridium perfringens* may be present after you cook foods; then while the foods are cooling down

Raw Meat: A Major Bacterial Danger

After you've finished handling raw meat, poultry, or seafood, put everything it contacted–knives, plates, and other utensils–directly into the dishwasher or sink, and don't use them again until they've been properly disinfected (see chapter 6 for more on food safety). Before handling any other food, wash your hands with antibacterial soap, particularly if your Risk Quotient is 3 or higher.

and before you store them in the refrigerator, these bacteria can multiply. Although institutional facilities (school cafeterias, nursing homes, prisons, hospitals) report the highest incidence of *C. perfringens*, they can still be present in your kitchen.

Signs and Symptoms: *C. perfringens* poisoning is usually characterized by sudden, painful intestinal cramps and diarrhea that begin from 8 to 22 hours after consumption of the bacteria.

E. coli

Where They Hide: *Escherichia coli* can be found on surfaces that have come into contact with uncooked or undercooked meat, unpasteurized milk and fruit juices, contaminated water or produce (like lettuce or alfalfa sprouts), and dirty hands. The most common household surfaces can host *E. coli*: kitchen sponges, kitchen and bathroom countertops, and the insides of sinks, bathtubs, and showers. You may also encounter *E. coli* on cooked foods that have picked up the bacteria from a contaminated kitchen surface, another food, or a serving dish (for example, a platter used to carry raw meats out to the barbeque that is later used to bring in cooked food without being cleaned).

Signs and Symptoms: Within 2 to 9 days after *E. coli* enters the body, you may feel severe abdominal cramps followed by diarrhea, nausea, and occasionally a low-grade fever.

Listeria monocytogenes

Where They Hide: Usually found on surfaces that have come into contact with milk, *Listeria monocytogenes* may also be found on leafy vegetables, processed meats, and unpasteurized dairy products, especially soft, unpasteurized cheeses. Common household surfaces include cheese cutting and serving boards, kitchen counters, and other kitchen utensils.

Signs and Symptoms: About a week after exposure, you may experience sudden flulike symptoms such as fever, headache, backache, abdominal pain, and diarrhea. *Listeria* infection is especially serious for high-risk individuals such as immune-compromised people, pregnant women, and the elderly.

Salmonella

Where They Hide: *Salmonella* is like *Campylobacter* in that it is easily spread in your home through cross-contamination, as when you cut raw meat and then use the same cutting board to chop vegetables. *Salmonella* can be found on any household surfaces that come into contact with raw and uncooked foods such as poultry, eggs, meat, seafood, unpasteurized milk, fruits, and vegetables. The most common household surfaces are cutting boards and kitchen counters.

Signs and Symptoms: About 6 to 48 hours after eating food with the *Salmonella* bacteria, you may have abdominal pain, diarrhea, nausea, chills, fever, and headache.

Staphylococcus aureus

Where They Hide: *Staphylococcus* bacteria, or staph, are spread by improper food handling practices and are found on your skin, in your throat and nose, and on kitchen surfaces that have come into contact with eggs, poultry, bakery products, and dairy products.

Signs and Symptoms: Within 30 minutes to 8 hours after eating staph-infected food, you may experience nausea, abdominal pain, and diarrhea often followed by weakness, fever, headache, dizziness, and chills.

Streptococcus pyogenes

Where They Hide: Eggs, milk, and shellfish that have been kept at room temperature for several hours before eating may contain strep bacteria, which can then contaminate kitchen counters, serving platters, and other dirty dishes.

Signs and Symptoms: Within 1 to 3 days after being exposed to strep bacteria, you may have an extremely sore throat, pain on swallowing, nausea or vomiting, headache, and a high fever.

Common Household Pathogens

Hepatitis A

Where They Hide: Many household surfaces can host other bacteria like the hepatitis A virus, which lurks particularly on kitchen counters, in vegetable bins, or on other surfaces that come into contact with lettuce, raspberries, strawberries, tomatoes, cold cuts, milk, and shellfish.

Signs and Symptoms: Hepatitis symptoms appear from 10 to 50 days after exposure and may last from 1 to 2 weeks. Symptoms may include fever and abdominal discomfort and may be followed several days later by jaundice.

Influenza

Where They Hide: The influenza A2 virus (and other variants of influenza) are spread by people who are already infected. The most common hot spots are surfaces that an infected person has touched and rooms where he has been recently, especially areas where he has been sneezing.

Signs and Symptoms: In just 1 to 3 days after you are exposed, you may experience a fever, headaches, congested nose, cough, and sore throat.

Rhinovirus

Where They Hide: The most common hot spots for rhinoviruses, typically the cause of common colds, are surfaces that an infected person has touched and rooms where she has recently been, especially if she has been sneezing.

Signs and Symptoms: About 1 to 3 days after exposure to the rhinovirus, you may have headaches, a sore throat, and a congested nose that can last for 7 days.

The Pros and Cons of Natural Cleaners

Since antibacterial products may upset the balance of microorganisms in and around us and may leave resistant germs behind, some scientists are advising us to take a step back in time to the cleaning products our mothers or grandmothers used, such as soap, hot water, chlorine bleach, ethyl alcohol (ethanol), hydrogen peroxide, and vinegar. With so many commercial cleaning products on the market today, you may wonder which ones work best.

In a study published in 2000 in the journal *Infection Control and Hospital Epidemiology*, researchers at the University of North Carolina, Chapel Hill, examined the effect of several commercial and natural disinfectants on disease-causing microbes including *Staphylococcus aureus*, *Salmonella choleraesuis*, *Escherichia coli* O157:H7, *Pseudomonas aeruginosa*, poliovirus, and vancomycin-susceptible and vancomycin-resistant *Enterococcus* species. The study found that the commercial products tested, including three hospital disinfectants (Vesphene IIse, TBQ, and ethanol) and four household disinfectants (Clorox bleach, Lysol Disinfectant Spray, Lysol Antibacterial Kitchen Cleaner, and Mr. Clean Ultra), were much more effective in killing these organisms than the two natural products tested (baking soda and vinegar). In fact, all of the commercial products were effective at completely inactivating the susceptible and resistant bacteria tested. Only bleach and Lysol Disinfectant killed poliovirus, the most rugged of the organisms tested.

To Sanitize or to Disinfect?

Sometimes it's enough just to *sanitize,* meaning to kill *most* germs and bacteria. Other times you want to *disinfect,* meaning to kill *all* germs and bacteria. A good rule of thumb is to always disinfect "hot spots," areas with high concentrations of dangerous germs—and a possibility that they might be spread to others.

However, while commercial products like bleach are highly effective, proven germ killers, they can contain strong chemicals and can irritate your hands, eyes, and lungs, and so some people prefer to use more natural alternatives in their homes. To offer you a range of options for cleaning your home, I'm including the recommendations of herbalist Laurel Vukovic, whose column "Home Remedies" has appeared in *Natural Health* magazine for more than a decade. Laurel's tips have encouraged and inspired many people to experiment with natural alternatives to commercial cleaning products.

You may find that some of these natural products will require you to clean more often. And because alternative products don't contain preservatives, you'll need to devote a little extra time to making up fresh batches before you clean. You may also wish to rotate between using commercial and natural products, for while it is important to stick with products that work, changing your cleaning tactics may also help reduce any long-term problems of breeding resistant organisms.

Let's take a look at some of these products, from the mild antimicrobial cleaners available at most natural foods stores to their more scientifically proven counterparts.

Alcohol

This disinfectant is traditionally used in the medical field to clean the skin and hands. Alcohol evaporates quickly and leaves no residue behind, making it an excellent choice for cleaning your telephone and computer keys, as long as it doesn't damage the plastics used to make these products.

Baking Soda

The chemical name of this cleaner/deodorizer is sodium bicarbonate. Use it to scrub shiny surfaces without scratching and to absorb odors in the refrigerator, sink drains, and garbage disposal. Baking soda also softens fabrics and removes certain stains.

Borax

This naturally occurring mineral is water soluble and can disinfect and deodorize. Use it to inhibit the growth of mildew and mold, to boost the cleaning power of soap or detergent, and to remove stains.

Chlorine Bleach

This relatively inexpensive and highly effective disinfectant kills most bacteria, including *Salmonella* and *E. coli*, which cause intestinal illness; *Staphylococcus*, which causes skin infections; rhinovirus, the leading cause of the common cold; and rotavirus, the major cause of diarrhea in young children. A good indication of how effectively it disinfects, bleach also killed more than 99.9 percent of the poliovirus microbe, a germ that is extremely difficult to destroy, in a 2000 study.

To clean with bleach, mix 1 tablespoon (to *sanitize*) to ¾ cup (to *disinfect*) liquid bleach with 1 gallon water. (See "To Sanitize or to Disin-

Bleach Warnings

Bleach is a strong chemical, so be sure to dilute it with water. Never inhale the fumes, as they may irritate your lungs. Do not combine bleach with other cleaners, such as ammonia, because dangerous chemical reactions may occur. Always keep bleach and other chemicals out of the reach of children.

fect?" on page 246.) After cleaning the area with soap and water to remove any surface grime, liberally apply bleach solution with a sponge, keeping the surface wet for at least 2 minutes; allow to air-dry without wiping. *Do not mix bleach and ammonia.*

Cornstarch

This foodstuff can be used dry, or it can be mixed with water to form a solution or paste to shampoo and deodorize carpets, clean windows, and polish furniture.

Essential Oils

Essential oils are aromatic liquids derived from plants. While they are known mainly because of their use in aromatherapy or massage, many of these oils have antibacterial, antiviral, and antifungal properties. Here are the essential oils discussed in this chapter, along with some suggested uses for them.

Eucalyptus. Eucalyptus is a potent antiseptic—that's why it's included in many household cleaning products and personal care products such as mouthwashes. *Eucalyptus globulus* has antibacterial and antiviral properties; the variety *E. citriodora* also has antifungal properties and a pleasant lemony scent.

Geranium. Geranium (*Pelargonium graveolens*) contains antiseptic and deodorizing properties; it has a strong citrus-rose scent that combines well with lavender, patchouli, and citrus oils. Try the following recipe for a wonderful smelling natural hand soap:

Geranium-Citrus Hand Soap

½ cup unscented liquid castile soap
10 drops geranium essential oil
10 drops lime essential oil
10 drops lavender essential oil

Mix the ingredients, shake them well, and pour into a pump-top dispenser.

Lavender. Lavender (*Lavandula angustifolia*) is effective against a wide range of bacteria, viruses, and fungi. It is gentle enough to use directly on the skin and is generally safe for children. Lavender blends well with other essential oils, and it softens the scent of medicinal smelling oils such as tea tree. It has a calming effect and is pleasant as an all-purpose oil for household cleaning.

Lime. Lime (*Citrus aurantifolia*) has general antiseptic properties and a refreshing, uplifting scent that can be used interchangeably with lemon essential oil.

Lemon. Lemon (*Citrus limon*) is a general, all-purpose antiseptic with a refreshing, energizing light scent. It is likely to cause skin irritation, so wear household gloves when using it in cleaning formulas.

Sweet orange. Sweet orange essential oil (*Citrus sinensis*) is an antibacterial and antifungal agent with a sweet, fruity scent. It works well in combination with patchouli oil. It may cause skin irritation, so wear household gloves when using products containing it.

Patchouli. The essential oil of patchouli (*Pogostemon cablin*) has antibacterial, antiviral, and antifungal properties. The rich, earthy, tenacious scent is excellent for eliminating odors in bathrooms, diaper pails, and the like. It also makes an effective natural hand soap.

Patchouli-Lavender Hand Soap

½ cup unscented liquid castile soap
25 drops lavender essential oil
10 drops patchouli essential oil

Mix the ingredients, shake them well, and pour into a pump-top dispenser.

Rosemary. Rosemary (*Rosmarinus officinalis*) has general antiseptic properties, and its use dates back to the Middle Ages when it was believed by some to protect against the plague. Its strong herbal and camphor scent combines well with lavender.

Tea tree. Tea tree (*Melaleuca alternifolia*) is a potent antiseptic and is effective against bacteria, fungi, and viruses. It is used in many commercial cleaning and disinfecting products and has a strong camphor scent.

Hydrogen Peroxide

A 3 percent solution may be an excellent sanitizer, especially when its use is followed by use of vinegar. Preliminary results of a 1996 study run at the University of Nebraska showed that pairing the two substances in mist form killed virtually all *Salmonella*, *Shigella*, and *E. coli* bacteria on contaminated surfaces—making this combination one that future studies might show to be as effective as chlorine bleach. Using two separate spray bottles, fill one with hydrogen peroxide and the other with plain white or apple cider vinegar. Spray the surface with one, allow to dry, then follow with the other.

Hydrogen peroxide also kills molds. Mix ½ cup hydrogen peroxide with 1 cup water in a spray bottle and spray on moldy areas in your home. Be careful about spraying hydrogen peroxide and vinegar since they can damage fabric and irritate eyes; also avoid breathing the spray.

Lemon Juice

The citric acid in lemon juice is a deodorant that can be used to clean glass and remove stains from aluminum and porcelain. Simply slice and squeeze a lemon and use the juice like bleach to lighten stains.

Lemon Oil Cleaner

Aromatherapists say that the scent of lemon boosts alertness, so use this fragrance in rooms where you need to be productive and alive. Lemon oil is antimicrobial and is used in many cleaning products. Add 9 drops lemon essential oil (*Citrus limon*) to 1 gallon water to clean floors.

Mineral Oils

These are effective ingredients in furniture polishes and floor waxes. Add 10 drops mineral oil to ⅛ cup vinegar for a natural cleaner and polish for wood furniture.

Orange Cleaner

This is a natural citrus cleaner available in natural foods stores. It's made from orange peels and removes dirt and grime without petroleum solvents. Use it to take off sticky labels or wipe down appliances, or to shine wood furniture, wiping off the residue as you clean. Remember to test it first to be sure it will not discolor the furniture.

Vinegar

Vinegar (acetic acid) is a mild acid that can dissolve mineral deposits and grease, remove traces of soap mildew and wax buildup, polish some metals, and deodorize. Use vinegar to shine windows without streaking. Also use vinegar in combination with baking soda to clean drains and garbage disposals—just be aware that the smell can be very powerful.

Water

Sometimes this is all you need—particularly if it's hot! When water is heated to 175° F for a sufficient period of time (from 5 to 10 minutes), it can inactivate most bacteria so they don't function properly. Some germs need higher temperatures than others to kill them, however, and there are some spores (bacteria in a dormant state) that survive even in boiling water—so it's wise to follow up with a disinfectant from time to time to ensure that the germs are gone. Don't try to clean with boiling water, since this can lead to severe burns. Instead, add ½ cup chlorine bleach to the hot water in your washing machine to kill bacteria. Or, add 2 tablespoons chlorine bleach to a sinkful of hot dishwater to keep germs from breeding.

Household Hot Spots: Your Virtual Germ Tour

Now that you know what pathogens lurk in your home and have an idea of some of the wide range of cleaning options you have to eradicate

> **Put On the Gloves**
>
> Always wear gloves when cleaning bacteria-laden surfaces; you'll protect your hands not only from germs but also from the irritating effects of the cleaning products.

them, it's time to get down to business. In this section I'll review each household hot spot—areas that need special attention—along with several safe solutions, plus my recommendations for custom-tailoring these techniques for your Risk Quotient. You'll see that I've tagged some problems with a Red Alert, to let you know these are known to harbor the greatest number of disease-causing bacteria and need special attention.

Culprits in the Kitchen

Appliances

Problem: Appliances are not as hospitable to bacteria as other kitchen surfaces because they are usually dry. Still, it's important to keep your appliances clean and disinfected, especially around handles where germs from our hands can easily be transmitted to others.

Solution: Use warm water and plain soap to scrub food and debris from appliances then follow up with a sanitizing or disinfectant solution. Pay special attention to handles. Wipe dry with paper towels.

RQ 1 RQ 2 Clean appliances whenever needed using the formula on page 254. Disinfect surfaces each month using 1 tablespoon bleach in 1 cup water.

Natural Antibacterial Cleaner

8 ounces unscented liquid dishwashing soap
2 tablespoons distilled white vinegar
20 drops lavender essential oil
20 drops lime essential oil

Combine the ingredients in a plastic bottle and shake well. This cleaner doubles as a terrific dish soap.

RQ 3 Clean appliances whenever needed using either the formula above or your preferred commercial cleaner. Every other week, disinfect surfaces using 1 tablespoon bleach in 1 cup water; wipe dry with paper towels.

RQ 4 **RQ 5** Clean appliances whenever needed using either the formula above or your preferred commercial cleaner; wipe dry with paper towels. Every other week, disinfect surfaces using 1 tablespoon bleach in 1 cup water. Leave the solution on appliances for at least 2 minutes to kill germs; wipe dry with paper towels.

Countertops

Problem: Because bacteria have a hard time surviving on dry surfaces, germs usually live for just a few hours on kitchen countertops. If you clean them frequently with contaminated sponges or dishrags or allow moisture to remain, this can promote bacterial growth.

Solution: Use ordinary dish soap, warm water, and a disinfected sponge or a paper towel to wash away any food debris from countertops. Periodically spray countertops with a sanitizing spray depending on your Risk Quotient. Allow the countertops to air-dry.

RQ 1 RQ 2 Use either your preferred commercial cleaner or the following spray to clean and sanitize your countertops weekly. After spraying the counter and allowing the solution to sit for a minute, dry the countertop completely with a clean paper towel.

Natural Antibacterial Spray

1 tablespoon borax
1 cup hot water
1 cup distilled white vinegar
½ teaspoon liquid dishwashing soap
½ teaspoon sweet orange essential oil
¼ teaspoon rosemary essential oil
¼ teaspoon lavender essential oil

Dissolve the borax in the hot water and allow the mixture to cool to room temperature. Pour the solution into a spray bottle, add the remaining ingredients, and shake well. The essential oils in this spray smell great, and this cleaner can also be used to sanitize telephones, computer keypads, and doorknobs.

RQ 3 Once weekly, spray your countertops alternately with hydrogen peroxide followed by vinegar, or clean with your preferred commercial cleaner.

RQ 4 RQ 5 Each day, if you use your countertops, wipe them clean. Every week, clean your countertops with either your preferred disinfecting cleaner or a solution of 1 tablespoon bleach in 1 cup water. Leave the solution on the counter for 2 minutes, then wipe dry with a paper towel. (Test this solution first to make sure it won't damage your countertops.)

RED ALERT

Cutting Boards

Problem: Cutting boards are a serious health concern because they are constantly exposed to raw meat, poultry, and seafood. When you make cuts into the board's surface, the tiny ridges that remain can become a breeding ground for dangerous bacteria.

Solution: Use two cutting boards—one for meats, poultry, and seafood, and the other for all other foods. While wooden cutting boards appear to ward off germs better, they are more difficult to disinfect because they warp in the dishwasher. Both plastic and wooden boards can and should be disinfected. After use, scrub the cutting board with ordinary dish detergent and hot water. Put your plastic cutting board into the dishwasher for a cycle. While research has been done on disinfecting wooden boards by placing them in the microwave, there are no safe guidelines on this practice—and it can present a fire hazard. Replace your wooden cutting board once the surface becomes clearly worn. Depending on your Risk Quotient, periodically rinse your cutting boards with a disinfectant solution, and allow them to air-dry.

RQ 1 RQ 2 Clean your cutting boards with hot, sudsy water following each use and allow them to air-dry. Whenever you prepare raw meat, use a plastic cutting board and wash it in the dishwasher after use. Use the following recipe to clean wooden cutting boards and butcher blocks:

Butcher Block Cleaner

¼ cup baking soda
2 tablespoons lemon juice

Mix the ingredients together and apply to butcher block surface with a clean, damp sponge. Let sit for 15 minutes. Scrub thoroughly, and rinse well with clean water.

RQ 3 Clean your cutting boards with hot, sudsy water following each use and allow them to air-dry. Place a plastic board into the dishwasher following each use. If you use a wooden cutting board, use a solution of 1 tablespoon bleach in 1 cup water to wipe down your boards. Rinse thoroughly and allow the boards to air-dry.

RQ 4 RQ 5 After cleaning your cutting boards thoroughly with hot sudsy water, sanitize them using a solution of 1 tablespoon bleach in 1 cup water after each use. Allow the bleach solution to stay on the board for 2 minutes to fully disinfect the boards, then rinse them thoroughly and allow them to air-dry.

Floors

Problem: Considering the multitude of raw foods that fall off cutting boards and countertops onto the kitchen floor, it's not surprising that kitchen floors often have a high bacteria count. While the good news is that most of us do not eat off our kitchen floors, good home hygiene dictates that we keep our kitchen clean. And anyone with young children needs to pay extra attention to all floor surfaces.

Solution: Sweep your floor frequently. Wipe up spills immediately, and mop the floor often to keep it sanitized.

RQ 1 RQ 2 RQ 3 Once weekly, use either your preferred commercial cleaner or the following sanitizing Kitchen Floor Cleaner:

Kitchen Floor Cleaner

2 gallons hot water
2 tablespoons liquid dishwashing soap
1 cup distilled white vinegar
10 drops rosemary essential oil
10 drops lavender essential oil

Mix the ingredients in a large bucket and stir the contents thoroughly. Use this solution to wash your floor using a mop or rag. Rinse with clean water.

RQ 4 RQ 5 Wipe up food spills immediately. Use the cleaner above or your preferred commercial cleaner twice weekly to keep the kitchen floor sanitized.

RED ALERT

Garbage Disposal

Problem: The garbage disposal is another hot spot for bacteria. Not only do food particles sit in the disposal day after day, but bacteria thrive in this moist environment. When you turn on the disposal, bacteria are dispersed into the air as aerosol particles that can contaminate everything in the vicinity.

Solution: If you have a sink stopper that fits over the drain, use it whenever you run the disposal to keep germs from flying up. Keep your disposal clear of food by rinsing it thoroughly after each use and flushing it with plenty of water. In addition, clean the disposal by pouring a sanitizing or disinfectant solution down the drain periodically. If you use the countertop Natural Antibacterial Spray (page 255), you might consider pouring it down the drain before you mix up a fresh batch.

RQ 1 RQ 2 Disinfect your garbage disposal each week using the following recipe:

Garbage Disposal Cleaner

- ½ cup baking soda
- 3 drops sweet orange essential oil
- ½ lemon rind

Mix the ingredients together and pour down the disposal. Run the disposal, using plenty of hot water to thoroughly rinse the drain.

RQ 3 Clean your disposal twice a week using the Garbage Disposal Cleaner above. Once weekly, pour 1 tablespoon bleach dissolved in 1 cup water into the disposal. Let it stand for 5 minutes, then run the disposal and rinse thoroughly with running water.

RQ 4 RQ 5 Clean your disposal twice a week with the Garbage Disposal Cleaner. Twice weekly, pour 1 tablespoon bleach dissolved in 1 cup water into the disposal. Let it stand for 5 minutes, then run the disposal and rinse thoroughly with running water.

Refrigerator

Problem: Spills of food on the refrigerator shelves and walls can lead to bacterial breeding grounds that call for attention.

Solution: Keep spills to a minimum and clean them up quickly using paper towels, soap, and water. Sanitize your entire refrigerator periodically—remove all food and place it into another fridge or cooler, discarding any outdated or spoiled items. Turn off the refrigerator and

A Fresh-Smelling Fridge

After you've cleaned the refrigerator, put a few drops of lemon or sweet orange essential oil on a cotton ball and tuck in the back of a shelf. The oil will keep your refrigerator smelling fresh until the next time you clean it.

unplug it. Take out all removable parts and wipe down the interior using a sanitizing or disinfectant solution. Wipe down all removable parts and the rubber around the door in the same way. Reassemble the refrigerator, plug it in, turn it on, and replace all food items.

RQ 1 RQ 2 Clean your refrigerator every 3 months using the following solution:

Refrigerator Cleaner

1 tablespoon baking soda
2 cups hot water
2 tablespoons distilled white vinegar
5 drops sweet orange essential oil

Dissolve the baking soda in the hot water. Add the vinegar and essential oil, and stir well. Wear rubber gloves, because orange essential oil can irritate your skin. Dip a sponge in the solution and wash the interior of the refrigerator. Rinse well with clean water.

RQ 3 Follow the instructions for RQs 1 and 2 to clean your refrigerator every other month. Clean up spills as soon as they occur and be conscientious about food storage and safety (see chapter 6).

RQ 4 **RQ 5** Clean your refrigerator monthly; first wipe down the interior and all parts using a solution of 2 tablespoons baking soda in 1 quart warm water. Then wipe down the entire fridge with a solution of ¾ cup bleach in 1 gallon warm water. Leave the solution on for 2 minutes to eradicate germs, then use paper towels to remove any remaining surface moisture.

RED ALERT

Sink

Problem: Scientists reveal that there is more fecal matter in a kitchen sink—which some call "the most germ-ridden spot in the home"—than in the toilet. *E. coli* can live on your hands for hours after you use the bathroom: If you neglect to wash your hands and later use the kitchen sink, that's where they will end up. This is especially frightening because children so often wash their hands at the sink before eating, or wash fruit for a snack. But when you think about it, the sink is the perfect breeding ground for germs—it is a moist area where contaminated food is frequently washed.

Solution: Rinse your sink thoroughly with clean, hot water after you have finished using it. If any residue remains, use a cleaner appropriate for your Risk Quotient. Be sure to sanitize the faucet, handles, and the back edge around the handles where the countertop stays damp.

RQ 1 **RQ 2** Clean your sink with ordinary soap and water at least twice a week. Once weekly, disinfect your sink using a mild bleach solution (1 tablespoon bleach to 1 cup water) or your preferred commercial cleaner. Use the following Drain Cleaner as needed:

Drain Cleaner

¼ cup baking soda
¼ cup borax
½ cup salt
½ cup distilled white vinegar
10 drops lemon essential oil

Mix the ingredients together and pour into the drain. Allow the solution to sit in the drain for 15 minutes, and then pour a teakettle of boiling water down the drain. Allow the water to cool completely before running the disposal again.

RQ 3 Keep your sink free of dirty dishes and standing water. Use a scouring cleanser to clean the sink every other day, followed by a bleach solution (1 tablespoon bleach in 1 cup water) or your preferred commercial cleaner. Use the above Drain Cleaner weekly, or more frequently if needed.

RQ 4 **RQ 5** Keep your sink free of dirty dishes and standing water. Disinfect your sink daily using either your preferred commercial cleaner or a solution of 1 tablespoon bleach in 1 cup water. Leave the bleach solution on these surfaces for 2 minutes to ensure that the germs are exterminated, then dry with a paper towel.

RED ALERT

Sponges, Dishcloths, and Dishtowels

Problem: Sponges and dishcloths are by far the most bacteria-laden objects in your kitchen. They are usually damp, and particles of food are embedded in them, giving bacteria everything they need to survive and multiply. In one study published in *Science News*, scientists grew enough *E. coli* and *Streptococcus* bacteria in a simple damp dishrag to cause serious illness.

Solution: Disinfect your sponge by running it with the dishes through a cycle in the dishwasher. Stock up on dishtowels; they should be changed frequently and laundered in hot water. If you prefer, disinfect your sponge by wetting and wringing it out, then placing it in the microwave on high for 1 minute. Remove the sponge using tongs and place it on a clean, dry countertop to cool. Be careful, as it will be hot! To disinfect a dishrag, wet it, wring it out thoroughly, spread it flat, and microwave it on high for 3 minutes. Carefully remove it using tongs, as it will be steamy hot, and place it on a clean, dry countertop to cool.

RQ 1 RQ 2 Disinfect sponges and dishcloths weekly by throwing them in your dishwasher. The hot water from the dishwasher, along with your regular detergent or this Natural Automatic Dishwashing Soap will work together to eliminate bacteria.

Natural Automatic Dishwashing Soap

2 tablespoons baking soda
2 tablespoons borax
2 drops lime essential oil

Mix the ingredients together and use entire amount in dishwasher.

RQ 3 Disinfect sponges and dishcloths twice weekly by using the microwave or dishwasher (see above). In addition, change dishtowels every other day to make sure the germs that breed overnight are not transferred to your hands or kitchen counters in the morning.

RQ 4 RQ 5 Disinfect sponges daily using the microwave or dishwasher (see above). In addition, avoid using dishtowels, opting instead for paper towels.

Bacteria in the Bathroom

Bathtub

Problem: Because the bathtub stays damp, it is a haven for bacteria as well as mold and mildew. Items left sitting on the sides of the tub, such as bars of soap, bottles of shampoo, washcloths, and loofah sponges, hold pools of water beneath them, adding to the bacterial hazards.

Solution: Clean your bathtub periodically using a cleaner appropriate for your Risk Quotient. A grout cleaner can remove stubborn stains and some mildew (follow directions). Buy wire racks for all your bath and shower products; they allow the water to drain from these items and reduce the amount of bacteria in the tub area. Toss washcloths and loofahs into the washer weekly and launder them in hot water.

RQ 1 RQ 2 Clean your bathtub every week using either your preferred commercial cleaner or one of the following cleaners:

Liquid Bathroom Cleaner

1 tablespoon baking soda
1 tablespoon borax
2 cups hot water
2 tablespoons distilled white vinegar
½ cup liquid dishwashing soap
20 drops eucalyptus essential oil
10 drops lavender essential oil
10 drops sweet orange essential oil

Dissolve the baking soda and borax in the hot water. Allow the mixture to cool to room temperature, and pour it into a plastic squeeze bottle along with the vinegar, dishwashing soap, and essential oils. Shake well. Apply the cleanser with a rag or sponge and rinse well with clean water.

Mold and Mildew Spray

- **2 tablespoons borax**
- **2 cups hot water**
- **¼ cup distilled white vinegar**
- **¾ teaspoon lavender essential oil**
- **¼ teaspoon tea tree essential oil**

Dissolve the borax in the hot water and cool to room temperature. Pour into a spray bottle, add the vinegar and essential oils, and shake well. To prevent mold and mildew growth, spray on surfaces and scrub with a soft brush. Rinse and allow to air-dry.

RQ 3 Clean your bathtub weekly, alternating between the bathroom cleaners above and these formulas: for the bathtub, use a solution of ½ cup bleach in 1 gallon water; for moldy areas, mix ½ cup hydrogen peroxide with 1 cup water in a spray bottle, and spray on liberally, followed up by spraying with either white or apple cider vinegar. Use caution in spraying both.

RQ 4 RQ 5 Clean your bathtub twice weekly using use a solution of ½ cup bleach with 1 gallon water. Clean moldy areas by mixing ½ cup hydrogen peroxide with 1 cup water in a spray bottle, followed up by spraying with either white or apple cider vinegar. Use caution in spraying both.

Floor

Problem: The bathroom floor might just be the dirtiest floor surface in your home. After all, the toilet sprays a host of bacteria onto the floor when it's flushed, the floor often remains fairly moist, and ongoing foot traffic in and out of this room carry in the germs your family has picked up at work and school.

Solution: Sweep your bathroom floor often to cut back on hair and other debris, and mop it frequently using a cleaner suitable for your Risk Quotient.

RQ 1 RQ 2 Sweep the floor at least once a week. Once weekly, use either your preferred commercial cleaner or the following one to keep germs at bay:

Bathroom Floor Cleaner

2 tablespoons borax
1 gallon hot water
1 teaspoon liquid dishwashing soap
5 drops patchouli essential oil
5 drops lavender essential oil

Dissolve the borax in the hot water. Add the soap and essential oils and mix well. Use a sponge or mop to wash the floor.

RQ 3 Sweep the bathroom floor twice weekly. Once each week, mop the floor using either your preferred commercial cleaner or ½ cup bleach in 1 gallon water. Allow the floor to air-dry.

RQ 4 RQ 5 Sweep the floor every other day to keep it clean. Once a week, mop the floor using either your preferred commercial cleaner or a disinfectant solution of ¾ cup bleach in 1 gallon water. Allow the floor to air-dry.

Shower Curtain

Problem: Bacteria love to hide in damp places, and most shower curtains are the perfect hosts. If you check your shower curtain thoroughly, you may see dark stains where it is wet or spots of soap residue or oils clinging to the sides. These are only temporary problems if you consider the following solution.

Solution: Open the shower curtain fully after showering to let it air-dry. Periodically wipe down the curtain with a sanitizing cleaner. Launder it occasionally using hot water and your favorite laundry soap plus ½ cup borax to disinfect and deodorize the curtain and to kill mold and mildew. Replace the curtain whenever it becomes worn or begins to tear. Consider washing your shower curtain periodically according to your Risk Quotient below.

RQ 1 RQ 2 Once a month, wash your curtain or use this tactic to rid your curtain of soap scum and residue:

Shower Curtain Cleaner

½ cup borax
½ cup distilled white vinegar
1 teaspoon liquid dishwashing soap
3 drops lavender essential oil
2 drops tea tree essential oil

Mix the ingredients together. Apply the solution to the shower curtain with a soft brush or sponge and scrub well. Rinse thoroughly with clean water.

RQ 3 Use the above solution every 2 weeks, followed up with Mold and Mildew Spray (see page 265).

RQ 4 RQ 5 Every 2 weeks, wipe your shower curtain thoroughly on both sides with a solution of ¾ cup bleach in 1 gallon water. Allow the curtain to air-dry. Follow up with this method for keeping mold and mildew at a minimum: Mix ½ cup hydrogen peroxide with 1 cup water in a spray bottle, and spray on liberally, followed up by spraying with either white or apple cider vinegar.

RED ALERT

Sink, Drain, and Faucets

Problem: Of all the problem areas in your bathroom, the sink, drain, and faucets are the real bacterial hot spots—the germs on your hands can spread to wet faucets when you turn them on, and as you scrub your hands or brush your teeth, bacteria cling to every damp spot they can find.

Solution: Wipe your bathroom sink periodically with a sanitizing or disinfectant solution to keep bacteria at bay. Pay special attention to the faucet, handles, and the area at the back of the sink that tends to remain damp. Also pay attention to mold or mildew in your bathroom, hiding underneath soap dishes or cups.

RQ 1 RQ 2 Once weekly, wipe the sink with either your preferred commercial cleaner or the following disinfectant:

All-Purpose Bathroom Disinfectant

2 cups warm water
¼ cup distilled white vinegar
½ teaspoon liquid dishwashing soap

- 10 drops patchouli essential oil
- 10 drops sweet orange essential oil
- 5 drops lemon essential oil

Mix the ingredients together in a spray bottle. Shake well, and spray liberally onto bathroom surfaces. Wipe with a clean, damp cloth or disinfected sponge.

RQ 3 Clean your sink weekly, alternating between the disinfectant above and either your preferred commercial cleaner or a solution of 1 tablespoon bleach in 1 cup water. Wipe dry with a paper towel.

RQ 4 **RQ 5** Disinfect the bathroom sink daily using either your preferred cleaner or a solution of 1 tablespoon bleach in 1 cup water. Let the solution stay on the surface for 2 minutes, then wipe it dry with a paper towel.

Toilet

Problem: Surprisingly, the toilet scores lowest on the hot spot list when it comes to germs, mainly because most of us are conscientious about keeping it disinfected. Bear in mind that each time the toilet is flushed, bacteria and viruses are propelled into the air and can land on any nearby surface—so store all personal care items far away from the toilet. Disinfect the handle frequently, as unwashed hands frequently make contact with it.

Solution: Periodically scrub the bowl and wipe down the entire toilet, including the seat and handle, with a sanitizing or disinfectant solution.

RQ 1 RQ 2 Sanitize your toilet weekly using either your preferred commercial cleaner or the following cleaner:

Toilet Bowl Cleaner

½ cup baking soda
½ cup borax
¼ cup distilled white vinegar
1 teaspoon liquid dishwashing soap
3 drops sweet orange essential oil
2 drops patchouli essential oil

Mix the ingredients together and pour into toilet bowl. Let sit for at least a couple of hours, and then scrub with a toilet brush and flush to rinse.

RQ 3 Clean your toilet bowl weekly, alternating between the cleaner above and either your preferred commercial cleaner or a solution of 1 tablespoon bleach in 1 cup water.

RQ 4 RQ 5 Disinfect your toilet bowl weekly using either your preferred commercial cleaner or a solution of 1 tablespoon bleach in 1 cup water. Apply the solution liberally and allow it to remain wet for 2 full minutes to kill bacteria.

Toothbrushes

Problem: It may surprise you—or sicken you—to know that if your toothbrush is stored near the toilet, the chances are great that it is covered with *E. coli* bacteria. Each time you flush the toilet, bacteria disperse into the air in the form of tiny aerosol particles that can land on any surfaces within 6 feet.

Solution: Keep the toilet lid closed when you flush. Store toothbrushes inside the medicine cabinet. Never share a toothbrush, as this can spread colds, the flu, and other infections including hepatitis B and C.

RQ 1 RQ 2 Replace your toothbrush cvcry 3 months.

RQ 3 Replace your toothbrush every 2 months.

RQ 4 RQ 5 Replace your toothbrush monthly.

Other Household Hot Spots

Computer Keyboard

Problem: The computer keyboard and mouse are two hands-on tools that host bacteria. Each time you use the computer after you sneeze or cough onto your hands—or simply touch your eyes, nose, or mouth—you've left your "mark." If you have a cold and a healthy person uses the computer after you, chances are great that these bacteria will find their way to the new host to invade and infect.

Solution: It's almost impossible to keep your computer keyboard and mouse germ-free, but you can periodically disinfect them. Turn the computer off, then pour a small amount of cleaning solution onto a paper towel, and gently wipe down the keys and mouse. You can also use a cotton ball or swab to clean between keys and get into other grooves. Be careful not to get any solution between the keys since they can be damaged, and remember—the best way to prevent the spread of germs is to encourage all users to wash their hands before and after they use the computer.

RQ 1 RQ 2 RQ 3 Clean the keyboard and mouse monthly using either the Natural Antibacterial Spray found on page 255 or your preferred commercial cleaner.

RQ 4 RQ 5 Clean the keyboard and mouse weekly using either alcohol or your preferred commercial cleaner. Wash your hands thoroughly before and after using the computer.

Doorknobs

Problem: Doorknobs, like telephone receivers, are perfect springboards for bacteria to jump from the hand of a sick person to the hand of a well person. And as soon as the well person puts a hand to his nose, eyes, or mouth, the germs have succeeded in infecting this new host.

Solution: It's not easy to keep doorknobs bacteria-free, but try to keep them as clean as possible by wiping with an antiseptic solution periodically. If someone in your family is ill with a cold or the flu, you should do this frequently. But remember, the best way to prevent infection is to wash your hands frequently and to insist that your family do so as well. Not every door requires you to touch the knob with your hand—many doors, including those in public rest rooms, can be pushed open using your shoulder or elbow.

RQ 1 RQ 2 RQ 3 Wipe doorknobs once each month using either the Natural Antibacterial Spray found on page 255 or your preferred commercial cleaner.

RQ 4 RQ 5 Wipe doorknobs twice a month with either rubbing alcohol or your preferred commercial cleaner.

Telephones

Problem: The telephone is another place where germs can spread from one person to another. Interestingly, most bacteria-related illnesses are transmitted by touching the handle or buttons—not the mouthpiece. When a sick person coughs or sneezes onto their hands, or simply touches her nose, eyes, or mouth, germs are spread to her hands. These infectious agents are then passed to the handle or buttons when a phone call is made. When the next unsuspecting person uses the phone, he picks up these germs—becoming the next host.

Solution: Periodically wipe your telephone receiver and buttons with a disinfectant, using either a cotton ball or swab. And remember—the main way to avoid picking up germs from the telephone is to wash your hands immediately after using it, especially when you're using a pay phone!

RQ 1 RQ 2 Wipe your telephone receiver and buttons every 2 weeks using either the Natural Antibacterial Spray found on page 255 or your preferred commercial cleaner.

RQ 3 Wipe your telephone receiver and buttons every week using either rubbing alcohol or your preferred commercial cleaner.

RQ 4 RQ 5 Wipe your phone twice each week using either your preferred commercial cleaner or a solution of 1 tablespoon bleach in 1 cup water. Wash your hands thoroughly after using the phone, and avoid public telephones if possible.

Washing Machine

Problem: Look no further than your washing machine for *E. coli* and *Salmonella*. For example, when you wash a load of your child's dirty undergarments, millions of fecal bacteria can spread to the next load. While *E. coli* will not survive a hot dryer, some other bacteria and viruses can.

Solution: Periodically add a sanitizing or disinfectant solution to the wash, and clean your washing machine using a solution based on your Risk Quotient.

RQ 1 **RQ 2** Use either your preferred commercial detergent or this Natural Laundry Detergent to clean and sanitize your clothing:

Natural Laundry Detergent

5 drops lavender essential oil
5 drops sweet orange essential oil
½ cup baking soda
½ cup borax
½ cup powdered castile soap

Add the essential oils by the drop to the baking soda and mix with a metal spoon. Put the mixture through a hand sifter to thoroughly distribute the oils. Add the borax and powdered soap and again sift well. Store in an airtight container. Add ½ cup to a full load of laundry.

RQ 3 In addition to using the Natural Laundry Detergent above or your preferred commercial detergent, add ½ cup bleach to the water when washing white undergarments, and use hot water. Disinfect your machine every 2 weeks by running it empty using hot water and adding ½ cup bleach to the water.

RQ 4 RQ 5 Add ½ cup bleach to the water when washing white undergarments, and use hot water. Disinfect your machine weekly by running it empty using hot water and adding ½ cup bleach to the water.

Outsmarting Bacteria

Clearly, there are many steps that you can take around your house to better manage germs. Targeted hygiene is simple—all you have to do is make sure there are no wet spots, and hit the known hot spots I've identified, to keep the bacterial risks in your home at a minimum. But remember that there will be times when you will need to be more vigilant. When a family member has a bacterial or viral infection, or when a visitor to your home has a high Risk Quotient, you'll need to take greater care to protect their health. For instance, if you are bringing home a new baby or if an elderly person is coming to stay with you, you'll need to disinfect the hot spots more frequently to further minimize the bacterial risks. You may also find that your lifestyle impacts the suggestions in this chapter: If you travel frequently and aren't home often, these recommendations may suggest too much cleaning; if have a very busy home with indoor pets, these guidelines may not be enough. Personalize your cleaning strategy to find what works for you.

6

EAT, DRINK, AND BE . . . WARY?

Imagine hosting a dinner party for close friends. Everything goes perfectly, and the menu is a complete success, from the melon balls with raspberries to the potato salad with feta cheese to the shrimp quiche. The next morning, however, you wake up feeling awful. You're vomiting, you have diarrhea, your body is aching, and you're running a slight fever. You wonder how you could have caught the flu—after all, it's the middle of summer!

The telephone rings, and as you walk to the next room to answer it, relentless intestinal cramps cause you to double over in pain. The caller, one of your guests from last night's party, says that he took his wife to the emergency room late last night, where she was diagnosed with food poisoning. As you hang up the phone, you mentally review your menu, wondering which food was the culprit. It could have been any of the items on your menu, as each of these protein-rich foods is commonly contaminated with bacteria: seafood, meats, poultry, eggs, and dairy products, as well as some fruits and vegetables including cantaloupe, raspberries, sprouts, and lettuce.

Experts say that reports of food-borne illness have increased over the past decade, partly because we've gotten better at identifying which diseases are actually caused by pathogens in our food. According to the Centers for Disease Control and Prevention (CDC) in Atlanta, food-borne pathogens cause more than 76 million of us—that's nearly one in every four Americans—each year to suffer from fever, stomach cramps, vomiting, and diarrhea. Complications such as jaundice, miscarriage, organ infections, meningitis, and respiratory arrest lead to 325,000 hospitalizations and 5,000 deaths. (While the estimated number of food-related deaths has decreased, this is still a significant number.) Those most susceptible to food poisoning include children under 5 (who are at risk of developing Hemolytic Uremic Syndrome [HUS], a condition leading to acute kidney failure), pregnant women, senior citizens, and anyone with compromised immune function. People with high Risk

Symptoms of Food-Borne Illness

Backache	Disorientation	Intestinal cramps
Chills	Dizziness	Lethargy
Constipation	Fatigue	Loss of appetite
Diarrhea (frequent, watery, sometimes bloody)	Fever	Nausea
	Headache	Vomiting

> **Report It!**
>
> If you or a family member suspect you may have gotten food poisoning, call your doctor and your local department of health. You should also contact the appropriate U.S. Department of Agriculture, Food and Drug Administration, or CDC hotline.

Quotients (RQ 4 or 5) may experience more drastic symptoms than those at lower RQs, but everyone is at risk. For low-RQ, generally healthy people, a food-borne illness can lead to a major, albeit temporary, disruption in their lives.

Even if you are conscientious, shopping in the cleanest grocery store, checking packaging for USDA labels and expiration dates, and watching for tears in boxes and dents in cans—all of which you should do—food still can become tainted even before it hits the shelves. During processing, fruits and vegetables may be handled by workers with poor hygiene habits, and the packing crates themselves can be contaminated. Also, long before food animals are butchered, they may have been fed contaminated feed, or they could have contracted infections that are harmful to humans from other animals held nearby in close quarters. This is an area where public health authorities have moved into the Age of Risk Management.

Antibiotics in Our Food: Weighing the Benefits

While there is little dispute that sick food animals should receive antibiotics to ensure a healthy livestock population, much debate is currently raging about whether treating healthy animals with antibiotics to make them grow faster and bigger is a good idea. The concern is that healthy animals can develop strains of resistant bacteria that might then be transferred to humans.

This problem has not been documented extensively, although Robert Tauxe, M.D., and his colleagues at the CDC, along with other independent researchers, have traced outbreaks of multidrug-resistant *Salmonella* to contaminated beef. And in a study published in 1999 in the *New England Journal of Medicine*, researchers found that chickens treated with a powerful family of antibiotics known as fluoroquinolones developed resistant *Campylobacter jejuni* bacteria (cause fever, diarrhea, and abdominal cramps in humans) that survived the period of treatment and, in many cases, up to the time of slaughter.

Clearly, the extreme position that antibiotics use in animals should be encouraged without restriction would lead to overkill. Nonetheless, the other extreme position—that antibiotics should never be used in animals—does not allow the important benefits of modern science and technology that we have come to depend on. The use of antibiotics in the production of food animals is now standard practice, and changes in that practice would alter not only the cost of production but also the

Foods to Avoid

If you have a Risk Quotient of 4 or 5, avoid these high-risk foods:

- Raw or undercooked meat, poultry, seafood, or eggs
- Processed meats (hot dogs, cold cuts)
- Unpasteurized milk and dairy products
- Feta, Brie, Camembert, and veined cheeses such as Roquefort
- Soft cheeses
- Unpasteurized or fresh-squeezed fruit or vegetable juices

risks. A sudden halt to the use of antibiotics might reduce the risk for certain resistant bacteria, for instance, while increasing the number of some other deadly pathogens. Currently, the Food and Drug Administration's Center for Veterinary Medicine is developing a process to manage these risks. Meanwhile, you can take important steps to significantly reduce the risks posed by the foods you eat.

Safe Food Storage, Preparation, and Cooking

Most food-borne illness is usually related to personal food handling practices, so the actions you take have a tremendous impact on your family's health. Using the Risk Quotient you determined in chapter 2, I will now take you through strategies to safely store, prepare, and cook your food.

Store Food Properly

Food is perishable—it goes bad when stored improperly. When you let cold food get warm or warm food get cold, you set the stage for disease-causing bacteria to multiply and infect you or your family members. Let the following rules alert you to potential problems with food storage so that you and your family can stay well:

Buy cold foods last. When shopping, pick up your packaged and canned foods first, and buy perishable foods such as milk, eggs, and meat at the end of your shopping trip.

Check the date. Check the expiration dates on all food labels, and never buy outdated food, even if it's on sale. Also check any "use by" stamps on dairy products (cheeses, sour cream, or yogurt). Pick the date that will last longest in your refrigerator, and make sure to use the foods by those dates. When you clean your refrigerator, check the dates on perishable items and toss any food that has an expired date.

Inspect carton contents. When it comes to eggs, don't stop at checking the expiration date. Open the carton and inspect each egg to make sure that there are no cracks in the shells—an ideal way for bacteria like *Salmonella* to enter.

Find the freshest catch. If you buy fresh fish, make sure the store's counters are clean and that the fish are lying on beds of ice. Ask the retailer about the freshness of the fish, and don't buy it if it smells strong. There is no odor in fresh fish!

Check precooked foods. If you buy cooked foods make sure that they are stored in separate containers from raw meats. If the employees working at the counter are also handling raw meats for customers, ask them to change their gloves before packing your order.

Examine produce carefully. Make sure salad greens are fresh and crisp, without any brown or slimy leaves.

Bag it! Grocery stores commonly offer plastic bags in the meat section, as well as in the produce aisle. Use the bags to wrap each meat package separately, as well as eggs, fruits, and vegetables. This will help

Produce Warning

Because fruits and vegetables are commonly contaminated with food-borne pathogens, be sure to wash them *thoroughly* before eating. The following list contains some produce particularly worth watching–and washing.

Alfalfa sprouts	Lettuce	Scallions
Basil	Potatoes	Strawberries
Cantaloupe	Raspberries	Tomatoes

to avoid cross-contamination, which occurs when bacteria from one food are carried to another food.

Keep it cool. Take all groceries home immediately so food does not spoil in your car. If you have other errands to run, bring along a cooler and store any perishable items there on the way home.

Know fridge facts. Cold temperatures are the key to preventing spoiling and reducing the risk of food-borne illness. Perishable foods should be stored at 40° F or colder. For long-term freezing, keep your freezer at 0° F. Keep eggs and dairy products off the refrigerator door shelves, as they are the warmest areas in the fridge. Don't defrost or marinate meats on the counter or in the sink—use the fridge or microwave.

Store it properly. For centuries, meat has been preserved using salt (sodium chloride). The practice continues today with meats such as beef jerky, hot dogs, and luncheon or deli meats. High concentrations of salt draw water out of bacterial cells, helping to destroy many of the agents that cause foods to spoil. Salt also gives processed meats more texture. Another form of salt, sodium nitrite, has been used for several decades to add flavor and color as well as to inhibit the growth of bacteria such as *Listeria*, which is commonly found in hot dogs and lunch meats as well as soft cheeses, raw meat, and unpasteurized milk. This bacterium can be deadly in large amounts, and while sodium nitrite retards its growth, it does not kill *Lysteria*. To avoid possible cross-contamination of other foods, all processed meats should be kept refrigerated in their original containers.

Wrap 'em up. Unless you'll be splitting them into freezer bags and cleaning thoroughly afterward, keep all raw meats, poultry, and fish in their original containers. Place them in the bottom drawer of your refrigerator to keep their juices isolated and avoid cross-contamination.

Don't let leftovers linger. Store leftovers as soon as possible, ideally in shallow, covered dishes within 1 hour of cooking. When warm food is stored in a deep container, it takes longer for the center of the food to cool. This creates an ideal growth environment for bacteria like *Clostridium perfringens*, which is the one of the most common causes of food-borne illnesses. Pathogens like *Clostridium* thrive in large batches of foods such as casseroles or soups, so reheat leftovers thoroughly to 165° F to avoid food-borne illness.

Turn down the doggie bag. Think about it—by the time you're ready to leave a restaurant, your leftover food has probably been sitting on the table for an hour. By the time you get it into the safe harbor of your refrigerator, bacteria have already started to grow. If you simply can't leave it behind, then be scrupulous—take the leftover food home *immediately*, refrigerate it until you're ready to reheat it to 165° F, and eat it within 24 hours.

Special precautions for high-risk individuals. If your Risk Quotient is 4 or 5, or if you are otherwise at high risk for food-borne illness due to a special situation or condition (see below and chapter 7), take these extra precautions with your food handling to protect your health:

- Always bring a cooler while shopping, and place frozen and perishable items inside when you load your car. At home, put those items away first.
- Most of us don't know how cold our refrigerators actually are, so buy a good thermometer that's easy to read and keep it toward the back of the refrigerator. Make sure your fridge is at 40° F or below.
- Put leftovers in the fridge the minute you've finished eating, and use a food thermometer when heating them up to be sure they've reached 165° F.

(continued on page 286)

Optimal Storage Temperatures

Food	Temp (°F)	Storage Time
Meats, Poultry, and Fish		
Beef, roasts, and steaks	40	3–5 days
	0	6–9 months
Beef, stew meat	40	3–4 days
	0	6–9 months
Beef, ground (raw)	40	1–2 days
	0	3–4 months
Beef, ground (packaged, frozen)	40	2–3 days
	0	3–4 months
Beef, ground (cooked)	40	3–4 days
	0	2–3 months
Pork roast	40	3–5 days
	0	4–6 months
Pork chops	40	3–5 days
	0	4–6 months
Ham (uncured)	40	3–5 days
	0	6 months
Ham (cured)	40	5–7 days
	0	3–4 months
Chicken (whole)	40	1–2 days
	0	9–12 months
Chicken (pieces)	40	1–2 days
	0	6–9 months
Turkey (whole)	40	1–2 days
	0	12 months

Food	Temp (°F)	Storage Time
Meats, Poultry, and Fish		
Turkey (pieces, cooked)	40 0	1–2 days 6 months
Fish, fresh	40 0	1–2 days 2–3 months
Fish, frozen	40 0	Use immediately 3–6 months
Fish, cooked	40 0	3–4 days 1 month
Dairy and Eggs		
Milk, (whole or skim) pasteurized	40 0	1–5 days beyond "sell by" date; use original container 3 months
Butter	40 0	2 weeks 6–9 months (if made from pasteurized cream)
Sour cream	40 0	2 weeks Do not freeze
Ice cream	40 0	Do not store in refrigerator 2–3 weeks (opened), 2 months (unopened)
Yogurt	40 0	7–10 days Do not freeze
Eggs	40 0	3–5 weeks 1 year (egg products)

• When eating out, be careful to choose restaurants with a reputation for freshness. Avoid eating any dish that contains meat, poultry, or fish that is not fully cooked—*no rare or medium-rare meals!*

Handle Food Safely

I've mentioned the importance of hand washing throughout this book as the best way to prevent bacterial and viral infections, and I'll say it again. We scientists know that this single practice could eliminate *half* of all food-borne bacterial infections. In study after study, scientists continue to reiterate how important it is to remove bacteria from your hands by rubbing them together with soap and warm water for 20 seconds, paying special attention to the areas between fingers, and rinsing and drying your hands thoroughly and properly. Improper hand washing can actually *spread* germs, so it's important to establish good hand washing habits.

Hand washing is especially important to avoid cross-contamination, resulting when pathogens are carried from one food to another. This is most dangerous when bacteria are transported from a food that is about to be cooked to one that's about to be eaten. For example, if you've handled raw chicken, then diced carrots for a salad, you're at risk of cross-contaminating the carrots with any bacteria from the chicken.

Here are other food handling tips to keep your food safe and avoid cross-contamination:

Thoroughly wash fruits and vegetables. The fruits and vegetables you buy in supermarkets and at produce stands may look clean, but they can contain a variety of pathogens as well as waxy substances that are applied to keep the skins intact or the residues of manure, pesticides, and herbicides. Since fruits and vegetables are usually eaten raw, it's critical that they be washed thoroughly to avoid food-borne illness.

Throw away the outer leaves of lettuces and other greens, as they tend to be the most contaminated. Soak the remaining greens in a large pot of water, replacing the water as often as needed until no grit remains behind. Wash the surfaces of firm fruits and vegetables such as apples, pears, and eggplants with a soft brush and a dilute solution of mild dishwashing soap, then rinse thoroughly. For fruits and vegetables that are fragile, such as berries or grapes, soak them in a bowl of water to which you've added a few drops of liquid dish soap. After 10 minutes, remove and rinse them thoroughly under the tap. Avoid using dishwashing soaps that contain antimicrobial agents for washing fruits—that's overkill.

Wash meat surfaces. Rinsing raw meat thoroughly with cold tap water will remove many surface bacteria. Dry the meat with paper towels and throw these away, along with the contaminated packaging.

Handle meats with care. As soon as you've finished handling meat, poultry, or seafood, place the contaminated cutting board and utensils in the dishwasher or sink, and don't use them again until you've disinfected them. Use paper towels to clean up any remaining juices and throw these away. Wash your hands thoroughly, and then disinfect the countertop before preparing other foods there.

Use two cutting boards. Use one board for meat products and the other for all other foods. This will help to eliminate cross-contamination that could make you or a family member ill.

Use separate utensils. Don't use the same knives or ladles for raw and cooked foods during cooking. You may have never considered this, but cross-contamination can occur when you use a fork to break up your browning beef and then use the same fork to stir the bean salad. Another common mistake is using the same plate for cooked meats that was used when the meats were raw.

Pack It Safe!

Keep your child safe from food-borne bacteria by taking these steps when packing school lunches:

- Buy your child an insulated lunch box or sack to keep foods at the right temperature.
- Use a refreezable ice pack to keep cold foods cold and a thermos to keep hot items hot.
- Each week, have your child wash the lunch box out with warm soapy water, then rinse it and let it air-dry; do this more frequently if needed.

Don't reuse marinades. Don't use that marinade as a sauce to serve with your cooked meat. It's swimming with bacteria! Pour the leftover portion down the drain and then disinfect your sink.

Special precautions for high-risk individuals. If your Risk Quotient is 4 or 5, or if you are otherwise at high risk for food-borne illness due to a special situation or condition (see below and chapter 7), take these extra precautions with your food handling to protect your health:

- Avoid handling raw meat if it's at all possible, and do not engage young children in cooking when raw meat is involved. If you do handle raw meats, then wash your hands thoroughly, perhaps using a nail brush. This is one occasion when I do recommend using an antibacterial soap to disinfect your hands and cooking items.
- Consider using a fruit-and-vegetable wash available at your local supermarket. While I don't feel these are necessary for those at low risk, some studies have found that they remove more bacteria than regular washing, and they may remove the waxes on the produce, which can improve taste.

• Avoid handling raw eggs, and never eat foods containing them unless you know that they've been pasteurized. If you do handle eggs, wash your hands with hot, soapy water before and afterward, and wash and sanitize utensils, equipment, and work surfaces afterward. This is another instance where I recommend using antibacterial soap. If you are making a dish that calls for raw eggs, such as Caesar salad, eggnog, or hollandaise sauce, use a pasteurized egg product found on your grocer's refrigerated shelves.

Cook Food Thoroughly

Food must be cooked until it reaches the right temperature (see "Safe Cooking Temperatures," below) to make sure that harmful bacteria are eliminated. These tips will ensure that your food is thoroughly cooked:

Safe Cooking Temperatures

Use a meat thermometer to determine the temperature of a food at its center while it is cooking. When the internal temperature below is reached, the bacteria throughout should have been killed.

Type of Food	Internal Temp (°F)
Beef, all cuts	160
Veal	145
Lamb	145
Pork, all cuts	160
Chicken	180
Turkey	180
Eggs	160
Reheated foods (all)	165

Easy Does It

Like a hot meal when you get home? Consider using a slow cooker, also called a Crock-Pot. This countertop appliance cooks foods slowly at a low temperature, usually between 170 and 280° F. Even though the temperature chart indicates higher temperatures for some meats, the direct heat from the slow cooker, the lengthy cooking time, and the steam that is locked in under the tightly covered lid all work together to keep harmful bacteria at bay. Be sure to follow the instructions that come with the pot regarding its safe use.

Don't believe your eyes. If you think the color of beef indicates "doneness," you're wrong. You can't trust your eyes—so purchase a meat thermometer and use it! The new "instant read" thermometers can give you a response in 15 seconds. You can find these thermometers at most grocery or kitchen supply stores. Insert the meat thermometer in the thickest part of the meat, away from any gristle, fat, or bones, to get the most accurate temperature. If the meat is irregular in size, insert it in several places to make sure it is hot enough throughout.

Pathogens love poultry! Poultry is a breeding ground for *Campylobacter* and *Salmonella*, and it takes a lot of heat to ensure that these pathogens are killed. Again, the best way to tell if poultry is cooked correctly is to test it with a meat thermometer. Insert the thermometer into the thickest part of the poultry, away from the fat and bone, to get the most accurate reading.

Pork is no exception! You must use caution when cooking pork, too. Never partially cook pork, then refrigerate and finish cooking it later, as the bacteria will not be destroyed. It's okay to start cooking pork in the microwave or oven and then immediately place it on the barbecue grill to finish the cooking process, but make sure that the internal temperature is hot enough by testing the thickest part of the pork with a meat thermometer. Even if the inside is pink, once it has reached this temperature, it is safe to eat. Make sure to eat leftovers within 3 days, and reheat them sufficiently to kill all bacteria they contain.

Use the 10-minute rule when cooking fish. The "10-minute rule" will help you avoid infection when you cook fish. Measure the fish you are baking at the thickest point. Bake it at 450° F for 10 minutes per inch of thickness. For instance, a 1-inch salmon steak should be baked for 5 minutes on one side, then turned over and baked for 5 minutes on the other side to be safe to eat. If you add sauce, this increases baking time; if the fish is frozen, double the baking time to 20 minutes per inch of thickness. If fish ever smells funny, looks bad, or has a slippery coating, toss it.

Eggs only look innocent. *Salmonella enteritidis* bacteria can survive on the outsides of eggshells, which is why eggs are sanitized before leaving the processing plant. Yet *Salmonella* can also exist inside the egg, as bacteria within the hen's ovary or oviduct enters the yolk and white before the shell forms. That's why even eggs that appear to be perfectly clean with unbroken shells may contain disease-causing *Salmonella* bacteria. To kill these pathogens, egg dishes must be cooked to 160° F.

Safe Seafood

While you may love raw oysters, if you have an RQ of 3, 4, or 5, consider switching to cooked shrimp or scallops instead. For high-risk people, eating raw oysters can cause serious illness or even death from a bacterium called *Vibrio vulnificus*, which occurs naturally in water.

Special precautions for high-risk individuals. If your Risk Quotient is 4 or 5, or if you are otherwise at high risk for food-borne illness due to a special situation or condition (see below and chapter 7), take these extra precautions with your food handling to protect your health:

- Avoid rare or undercooked meat. Add 5 degrees to the temperatures shown in "Safe Cooking Temperatures" on page 289. The longer cooking time will kill more bacteria, which may help to protect your health in the long run
- Cook your eggs thoroughly. Moist scrambled eggs and soft-boiled eggs are off-limits. If you enjoy drinks with raw eggs like eggnog, use the store-bought variety and make sure the product you buy is pasteurized—that means it's been heated to a temperature that kills the bacteria contained in the eggs
- Whenever you're traveling, always carry your own bottle of water and a nutritious, filling snack. In the event you visit a restaurant where you're unsure about the food, you'll have a back-up plan to tide you over.
- If you attend a potluck supper or a party where several people have brought food, avoid any items that have been prepared by people who have recently been sick. Also avoid warm casseroles or creamy cold salads that may have been sitting out for a while, allowing bacteria to breed.

10 Common Food Safety Mistakes

Most food safety mistakes are made innocently, simply because we didn't know the rules. And with so many of us juggling multiple responsibilities at work and home, it's no wonder that we are more concerned with convenience and saving time than we are with washing that head of lettuce thoroughly before using it or heating up the leftovers to the proper temperature. That's why I've identified these food safety mistakes and their solutions—to show you how simple it can be to improve your food hygiene habits and reduce the risk of food-borne illness.

Mistake #1: Assuming that "prewashed" fruits and vegetables are really clean and ready-to-eat.

Solution: Wash *all* fruits and vegetables thoroughly before eating and cooking, even the ones that say they have already been triple-washed.

Mistake #2: Thinking a hamburger is done because it tastes fresh or "looks" done.

Solution: Appearances can be deceiving! Don't rely on your senses to tell you whether a food is cooked properly or has gone bad due to poor refrigeration. While you should avoid any foods that are visibly bad, you cannot always see, smell, or taste disease-causing bacteria. That juicy hamburger may appear to be well-done, but you cannot tell for sure by its color. Use the thermometer test and make sure it is cooked through to at least 160° F.

Mistake #3: Putting the grilled meat back on the same plate after you finish cooking or grilling it.

Solution: Never use the same plate to serve cooked meat that you used when it was raw. Place the dirty plate and utensils into the sink or dishwasher, and use fresh ones for the cooked meat.

Mistake #4: Tasting homemade cookie dough or cake batter that contains raw eggs. (After all, a little bite won't hurt anyone!)

Solution: It's true that a little taste probably won't hurt you, but one innocent bite often turns into several more bites, and each bite may host *Salmonella*, resulting in days of intestinal cramps, diarrhea, and suffering. Make sure your kids know this rule, too, and forego the traditional reward of letting them lick the spoon. By the way, ready-made cookie dough generally does not contain a risk of *Salmonella* because it is made with pasteurized eggs, which have been heated sufficiently to kill bacteria.

Mistake #5: Using the same dishtowel to wipe your hands and the counters.

Solution: This common mistake causes cross-contamination. Instead, wash your hands frequently with soap and water, then dry them on a clean paper towel. Keep a large supply of dishtowels on hand, and launder them frequently in hot water. Use paper towels to wipe the countertop and discard these after use.

Mistake #6: Stuffing a chicken or turkey hours before cooking.

Solution: Stuff the bird right before it goes into the hot oven. Letting time lapse between stuffing and cooking can allow bacteria to breed. In addition to testing the temperature of the poultry, test the temperature of the stuffing to make sure it reaches 165° F. Be sure to refrigerate uneaten stuffing soon after cooking to keep bacteria from growing.

Mistake #7: Eating cheese with mold on it, or other old food.

Solution: Many people delight in adding bleu cheese, whether Roquefort or Gorgonzola, to a fresh vegetable salad. This gourmet cheese is marbled with bluish or greenish veins of mold. While this mold is safe to eat, mold found on other cheeses (or any other food, for that matter) is a sign that it is going bad. If the cheese is hard, such as cheddar, and you see a small amount of blue, green, or white mold, simply cut it off. If the cheese is soft, toss it.

Mistake #8: Eating unwashed fruits.

Solution: More and more food-borne bacteria are found in fresh fruits and vegetables, particularly those that are shipped to the United States from overseas. Each piece of produce should be washed thoroughly. Produce with firm skins should be cleaned with a brush; more delicate fruits such as berries should be soaked and rinsed.

Mistake #9: Eating foods packed in dented or bulging cans.

Solution: If the can isn't in perfect condition, don't buy it. If you discover the problem after you get home, return it to the store or throw it away. Dents and bulges in cans are signs that something may have gone wrong in the process of packing or transporting it, and it could contain toxins released by the bacterium *Clostridium botulinum*. Even the tiniest amount of these toxins can kill you (on average, five people die of botulism each year), and normal cooking will not eliminate the toxin.

Mistake #10: Throwing suspect food away after eating some of it.

Solution: If you eat something and become ill, *always keep the evidence*. In order to avoid anyone else getting sick from the same food, wrap up the remains securely, mark them "Contaminated—Do Not Eat," and put them in the refrigerator. If you suspect food poisoning, write down the foods you ate, the dates and times that you ate them, and any symptoms you experienced. You may need this evidence later on if a food-borne pathogen caused a serious illness. If you have a Risk Quotient of 3 to 5 and suspect food poisoning, *seek immediate medical care*. If you served the food to others, call them to let them know you're ill and ask whether they have any symptoms. If you can't quickly contact everyone who ate the food, then notify your local health department to report a possible contamination.

A Word about Water

Even though you can't see them, bacteria can also be found in your drinking water. The U.S. Environmental Protection Agency (EPA) mandates that all water supplies be filtered, treated with chlorine, and tested regularly for the presence of fecal coliform bacteria. In general, bottled water is subject to the same standards as tap water. However, a study published in the journal *Epidemiology* suggests that, despite the EPA's regulations, drinking tap water may increase the incidence of gastrointestinal illness. While bacteria like *E. coli* may cause only minor symptoms for most of us, they could result in death for high-risk populations like infants, the elderly, and those with compromised immune function.

There are a variety of methods that can improve water quality:

• Water filters reduce the amount of sediment, dirt, debris, rust, and iron particles from the water. Carbon filters, such as those found in Brita water pitchers, can improve taste and odor and can filter certain contaminants from the water, but they do not remove bacteria or dissolved minerals.

• Water distillation uses heat to remove virtually all contaminants, including bacteria and sediment, from water. Bottled distilled water (not to be confused with spring water) is a safe alternative to distilling it yourself. Countertop distillation machines, similar to coffee makers in size, are available for around $400.

• Water softeners are used to reduce scale, a residue that impedes the performance of many household appliances. Water softeners work by removing the minerals calcium and magnesium, but they add sodium to the water, so check with your doctor if you're on a low-sodium diet.

• Reverse osmosis uses a pre-filter to remove sediment, a carbon filter to remove contaminants, tastes, and odors, and a membrane through which pressurized water flows to remove more particles. While this system removes bacteria, it may not kill them unless properly used. If the filter is old or dirty, it can even *add* bacteria to the water you drink.

• Disinfection is usually used in wells. This method relies on shock chlorination, in which a strong solution of chlorine is introduced throughout the entire plumbing system to kill bacteria and viruses.

While these methods can result in cleaner water, those with low Risk Quotients (RQs 1 through 3) may tolerate tap water with no problem at all. Those at higher risk should consider taking steps to reduce the amount of bacteria in their drinking water. If you have a Risk Quotient of 4 or 5, consider bottled distilled water, a countertop distillation machine, or the alternative of drinking only boiled water. Bring a pan of water to a full, rolling boil for 3 full minutes, then allow it to cool. Use this water for all your drinking purposes, including adding it to concentrated juices, brushing your teeth, and using it to make ice cubes.

What about Irradiation?

One controversial food safety technique is the use of *irradiation*, which destroys pathogens in food without making the food radioactive. For decades, the military has relied on irradiated foods to protect servicemen from food-borne illness, and irradiated meats are now commercially available in the United States. The FDA requires that manufacturers label irradiated foods with either "treated with radiation" or "treated by irradiation" and a radura, the international symbol for irradiation. While irradiation renders food safer by killing bacteria, some opponents believe that it could lead to relaxed sanitary procedures in food processing facilities.

While questions have been raised, research suggests that irradiating meats and poultry can significantly reduce the amounts of pathogens without reducing their nutritional value. It remains unclear whether consumers will come to accept irradiation as standard. If so, this practice could possibly yield a tremendous public health benefit, no matter what your Risk Quotient.

You Are What You Eat . . .

We must all eat to survive, though our food choices differ according to our preferences and the types of foods available to us. In this age of increased globalization, it's important to remember that locally grown foods are probably the freshest. Although technological developments in food processing and importing have made certain foods available year-round, they can lead to the introduction of new bacteria into your body—both good and bad bacteria.

In the long run, the evidence suggests that those people who eat a diverse diet, including a variety of locally grown and imported foods, and who consequently expose themselves to the broadest range of bacteria in small amounts, tend to have the least risk for bacterial illness. So go ahead: Eat, drink, and be *merry*—just as long as you're also *wary*, keeping your food as safe as possible using all my strategies for storing, handling, and cooking.

7

STRATEGIES FOR SPECIAL SITUATIONS

A variety of situations and circumstances automatically place you or your loved ones at a heightened risk for bacterial infection. Infants, young children, older people, and those with poor immune function should always take additional health precautions, as should those who spend any time in crowded quarters such as day care centers, dormitories, barracks, long-term care facilities, and hospitals. When you travel, too, you are likely to encounter germs with which your immune system is unfamiliar, and you should take steps to limit your exposure to these bacteria.

Protecting Your Children

If you or a family member is at high risk, then staying healthy is important so that you can help protect your child from experiencing undue risk. Let's look at the kinds of precautions you can and should take to keep your vulnerable young ones well.

Newborns

When babies are born, their immune systems are functionally immature, leaving them at high risk for infection the first 4 to 6 weeks of life. While newborns get some immune protection from the antibodies they receive from the placenta before birth and through the mother's breast milk (if breastfed), there are many germs that infants cannot produce antibodies against. It's important, therefore, to take steps to help newborns stay well, such as:

- Have your newborn room with you. This common practice while still in the hospital reduces the handling of your baby by others. Always wash your hands for 30 seconds before and after handling your baby, and dispose of soiled diapers in the appropriate place. Make sure anyone who comes to visit washes his or her hands before touching or holding the baby.

- Breastfeed your baby, which helps to build a strong immune system. Breast milk contains immune- and growth-building substances that are not contained in formula, and the composition of your milk changes as the child grows. It is most important to keep in mind, however, that your newborn needs adequate food and water, so talk to your pediatrician immediately if you have difficulty with breastfeeding or suspect jaundice. With the increase in breastfeeding and the trend of hospitals releasing mothers and their new babies before breastfeeding has been fully established, several cases of severe jaundice leading to permanent brain damage have been reported. Be sure to wash your hands thoroughly before and after breastfeeding; in addition, care for your breasts and keep them clean. If you are pumping breast milk, refrigerate or

The Pros of Breastfeeding

In a study reported in the *American Journal of Public Health*, babies who received only breast milk during their first 6 months experienced up to 30 percent fewer illnesses than their formula-fed counterparts. To take full advantage of this natural risk-reducer, the American Academy of Pediatrics recommends nursing for as long as possible, at least 6 months to a year.

freeze it immediately. Wash the pump thoroughly using warm water and soap as recommended, and allow it to air-dry. Keep breast milk cold until you are ready to feed your baby; then warm it and use it right away, before bacteria can multiply to dangerous levels. After feeding, discard any unused milk.

- If you bottle-feed your baby, sterilize bottles and nipples between uses either by running them through the dishwasher or by boiling them. After each feeding, discard any unused formula; germs from the baby's saliva will multiply quickly in it. Keep formula in the refrigerator until just before feeding time, then warm it and feed it to your baby immediately.

- Circumcision has become a complicated matter for today's parents, who must consider their own religious and cultural values as well as a host of conflicting health reports. Some studies find slightly increased instances of urinary tract infection and transmission of sexually transmitted diseases in uncircumcised males; many authorities, however, including the American Academy of Pediatrics, say that these findings are not conclusive enough to recommend circumcision. If you decide to circumcise your son, discuss the decision with your pediatrician beforehand, and ask for specific instructions on minimizing the risk of post-surgical infection. If you decide not to circumcise, keep his foreskin especially clean, washing it at bath time and during diaper changes. As he grows older, encourage him to cleanse his foreskin thoroughly while bathing or showering.

Babies and Toddlers

Young children do ongoing battle with viruses and germs as their immune systems develop. It's not abnormal for a preschooler to get six to eight colds each year or to have many bouts of ear infections, especially if they are in close contact with other young children. When a child has a weak immune system, she is even more susceptible to illness; here then are some proactive steps you can take to help keep your child well:

- Thoroughly wash any toys that your young child places in her mouth. While mouthing of objects is your baby's way of exploring the world, you will need to watch out for any items that might harbor bacteria in addition to any that are dangerous. Wash them with soap and water, allowing them to air-dry, or place plastic toys in the dishwasher.
- Keep your floors and other surfaces clean, as most babies will pick up items from the floor and place them into their mouths. Clean up any spilled or dropped food immediately, since these may harbor bacteria and may be of particular interest to your child as a possible food item.
- Wash your baby's pacifier with soap and water periodically, especially when he drops it onto the floor. Keep several pacifiers on hand so that you can give your baby a clean one while you wash and air-dry the others.
- Frequently wash your baby's hands with a clean washcloth and warm water, as babies love to put their hands into their mouths. Keep a small bottle of clean drinking water in your diaper bag so that you can keep baby's hands clean or rinse a dropped toy or pacifier when you're away from home.

• Replace your child's toothbrush regularly and keep family toothbrushes separate, particularly when someone in the family gets ill.

Day Care Facilities

Because children who spend time in daycare facilities are at higher risk for contracting bacterial and viral infections, parents must take extra precautions to ensure their child's health and safety. Consider these strategies:

• Use the criteria for selecting a childcare center outlined starting on page 181.

• Teach your child the importance of hand washing—and teach by example! Use the suggestions on page 188 to make hand washing a fun time so that he or she will embrace this critical hygiene habit.

• Keep your child at home when he is ill (following the guidelines in "Is Your Child Too Sick for Day Care?" on page 182) and make sure that your day care center enforces this policy. Otherwise, your child and in turn your entire family will be constantly exposed to "bad" germs.

• Be certain your child gets adequate sleep, a varied and nutritious diet, and plenty of time to play outdoors. If your child is a picky eater, ask your pediatrician about vitamin and mineral supplementation.

• Schedule regular "well child" checkups, and keep vaccinations and immunizations current. As I discussed earlier, this practice has virtually eradicated a number of infectious diseases, leading many parents to believe that vaccinations are no longer necessary. Without them, however, your child is left extremely vulnerable. If she has a chronic illness, such as asthma, ask your pediatrician about whether a flu shot is advisable (be sure to mention any egg allergies). Also, if your child is frequently ill or prone to ear infections, ask your pediatrician about whether the pneumococcal vaccine, which is now being recommended for children with chronic illnesses, is right for your child.

Close Quarters

College dorms and other crowded living environments are germ havens—people living together in a tight space, breathing the same air, touching the same surfaces, and therefore sharing the same germs. In fact, some frightening new studies reported by the Centers for Disease Control and Prevention (CDC) in Atlanta reveal that college freshmen living in dormitories have more than six times greater a risk of getting bacterial meningitis than other college students. Other risk factors for those in dorms may include such lifestyle habits as kissing, sharing drinks, engaging in sex, smoking, and binge drinking.

If you or a loved one will be living in a dorm or other close quarters, consider the following safe strategies to avoid infection:

- Wash your hands frequently and thoroughly to prevent the spread of bacteria. A 2001 article in the *American Journal of Preventive Medicine* described a program entitled "Operation Stop Cough" initiated at the Recruit Training Command Center in Great Lakes, Illinois. As part of this program, Navy recruits were instructed to wash their hands at least five times a day. Researchers found that the overall rate of respiratory illness decreased by 45 percent.

- Keep your immune system working at its peak by getting plenty of sleep, eating a nutritious diet, and avoiding stress. While this is not easy to do in a college dorm, schedule time for naps, especially if you are staying up late studying. Keep fresh fruits and vegetables for snacks in your dorm refrigerator, and make sure to wash them thoroughly before eating. And don't take on more extracurricular activities than you can handle—chronic stress is a known immune buster.

- When you go to the infirmary for a sore throat or other illness, question the prescribing doctor before taking antibiotics. Ask if the medication is absolutely necessary—meaning your infection is bacterial, not viral—and if you need antibiotics, make sure to take them exactly as prescribed.

- Get a flu shot. Most college campuses have inexpensive flu vaccines available for students and faculty members right after school starts in the fall. If you are allergic to eggs, specifically ask whether the vaccine is safe for you.
- A vaccine for bacterial meningitis is now available, and the American Academy of Pediatrics recommends that college students receive this immunization. Ask your family doctor whether this vaccination might be right for you.

Travelers

Even those with a low or moderate Risk Quotient are in jeopardy of getting a bacterial infection while traveling. Before your feet hit the ground of your destination, you may have been sitting in a crowded airplane with recirculated, bacteria- or virus-laden air, perhaps even seated next to a passenger who is clearly ill (in which case you should move if at all possible). Once at your destination, you're faced with food and water that may be contaminated. Infection with *E. coli* is responsible for between one-fourth and one-half of all cases of travelers' diarrhea in Jamaica and Mexico. Even if you travel to a country with excellent sanitation, you may experience gastrointestinal illness due to bacteria that are simply unfamiliar to your immune system.

Prevention is the best medicine, so use these tips to avoid illness while traveling:

- Plan ahead—get enough rest, eat well, and drink plenty of water for several days prior to your departure.
- If you're traveling overseas, get all of the recommended immu-

nizations at least 3 weeks before you leave. (If your health is poor, certain vaccines might not be appropriate for you. Talk to your doctor about this ahead of travel time.)

• If you are flying, arrive at the airport well ahead of time to avoid the stress of rushing. Bring along bottled water to drink while waiting for your plane—hydration helps your immune system to work at its peak. Also bring something relaxing like a book or magazine to read while waiting.

• While you're in the air, avoid diuretics like alcohol and caffeine. Opt instead for fruit juices and bottled water.

• If you're traveling in a foreign country, drink bottled water. Use only bottled or boiled water for drinking and when brushing your teeth if possible. If that is not possible, ask your pharmacist about a disinfectant agent, usually in tablet form, available at most pharmacies. In some countries, filtering or boiling water is also necessary to remove other debris and parasites.

• Beverages such as hot tea or coffee are usually safe to drink, but ask if the water has been boiled. Do not use ice cubes made from the local tap water.

• Ask your pharmacist about bringing oral rehydrational salts (ORS), a simple combination of salt and sugar available in portable sachet packages, to help prevent dehydration in case you get "traveler's diarrhea." Added to disinfected water, the ORS replenish vital salts and electrolytes and are recommended for overseas travelers by the World Health Organization.

• Avoid vegetables and fruits that cannot be peeled, as they may contain bacteria from the area's tap water. Don't be tempted to pick and eat fresh fruits and vegetables in foreign countries.

• Make sure that your meals are well-cooked and served hot. Food that is merely warm may have sat on a counter for several hours before reaching you, providing the perfect environment for breeding bacteria.

- Avoid dishes containing raw eggs such as Caesar salad or Hollandaise sauce and local dishes containing raw seafood, poultry, or meat. If you aren't sure what's in a dish, ask!
- Always wear footwear to avoid foot injuries, insect bites, and infections.
- Avoid swimming in freshwater ponds, rivers, streams, and lakes to avoid bacterial infections. Also be aware of any possible ocean hazards, like fecal contamination, that may make swimming risky. Make sure to ask—do not assume that just because you see local people swimming in the water that it won't make you sick; heed any health warnings, even if other people are not doing so.

Immune-Compromised People

Antibacterial resistance is an especially dangerous problem for people with impaired immune systems, such as those with AIDS, cancer patients undergoing chemotherapy, and people on immunosuppressive therapy, such as organ transplant recipients. Remarkably, approximately 90 percent of AIDS patients who acquire multidrug-resistant tuberculosis die as a result of the disease.

There are several strategies you can adopt to protect the health of those with impaired immune functions:

- Consider flu and pneumonia vaccines for all family members to prevent spreading illness to the individual.
- Provide a varied, nutritious diet for immune-compromised people. Make sure all food is thoroughly washed, well-cooked, and served at the appropriate temperature immediately after it's prepared. Pay special

attention to those foods noted for their antioxidant properties (see "The Antioxidant Success Story" on page 69).

- Ensure plenty of rest and relaxation.
- Use the hygiene recommendations in chapter 5, paying special attention to household hot spots. In any areas where the ill person will spend time, such as the bathroom, use the recommendations for the highest Risk Quotients (RQ 4 and RQ 5).
- Keep any medical devices, such as feeding tubes and syringes, sterilized and out of the reach of children.
- Ask the physician about any important food restrictions and whether the immune-compromised person should be drinking bottled, distilled, or boiled water.

Hospital Patients

There's no doubt that hospitals save millions of lives each year, but they also serve as hubs for the formation and transmission of drug-resistant bacteria. Approximately two million Americans acquire infections in hospitals each year, and more than half of these infections are resistant to at least one antibiotic. Today, experts estimate that up to one-third of hospital patients require antibiotics to fight or prevent infections—but these infections still cause over 19,000 deaths each year, constituting the 11th leading cause of death in the United States.

Although emergency hospitalizations do occur, many hospital stays are anticipated. If you're able to select your hospital, you can learn more about and perhaps tour it beforehand to get an impression of its cleanliness. In any case, here are a few actions that can help you stay infection-free:

- If possible, check out the cleanliness of the hospital ahead of time. Visit patient rooms, talk to others who have been treated there, and ask professionals you trust about the facility's reputation, including your doctors and other health care practitioners.

• Ask for a copy of the hospital's guidelines for avoiding hospital-acquired infections. Ask all personnel to abide by these rules when caring for you.

• Ask about the hospital's infection rate, including how many resistant bacterial infections they have had, the most recent infection, how many people were infected, and how frequently personnel are tested for pathogens. While this information may not be available, asking for it may help you understand how the hospital deals with the issue.

• Make sure that anyone in the hospital who treats you or your family member has short, natural fingernails, or, if not, is wearing gloves. In a study reported in the *New England Journal of Medicine*, researchers reported that pathogens were found more frequently on medical personnel wearing artificial nails. It's hard to know whether the person caring for you has real nails, but you can politely ask whether she has washed her hands or ask her to put on clean gloves before seeing you.

• With fewer than 50 percent of physicians and nurses washing their hands properly between patients, one study reported health care workers' tendency to overestimate their hand washing compliance. If someone comes into your room with gloves on, they should remove them, wash their hands thoroughly, and put on clean, sterile gloves before examining you or administering any treatment. If they don't do so, remind them!

• Wash your hands thoroughly after using the bathroom and after touching the sink, shower, or other damp areas in the hospital room. Other bacteria breeding grounds include incubators, respiratory-therapy equipment, and hand lotions used by staff members, contaminated when the bottle opening touches hundreds of people's hands each day.

• Wash your hands before and after eating your meals. Order your food well-cooked. When it arrives, it should be served at the appropriate temperature—hot foods hot, and cold foods cold—or notify your nurse and ask for another plate. Wash any fresh fruits or uncooked vegetables from the hospital's kitchen before eating them.

Older Adults

No one escapes the changes that come with age. You may find that you are more susceptible to bacterial and viral infectious as you grow older, and you may also find it more difficult to get over an infection. Older adults also need to use caution in taking any type of drug; their liver and kidneys cannot process drugs as quickly as younger adults, and this may create a greater threat of adverse or toxic drug reactions and drug overdoses.

Because aging adults need to be so cautious about bacterial and viral infections, consider the following strategies:

- Keep your immunizations up-to-date. Talk with your doctor about influenza and pneumonia vaccines to determine if they are right for you.
- Eat a healthful diet, get sufficient exercise, drink lots of water, and get plenty of rest to keep your immune system functioning optimally.
- Wash your hands thoroughly several times a day—upon rising, before and after preparing food, before and after eating, and after using the bathroom. Many infectious diseases are transmitted by touch, and thorough hand washing can significantly reduce your risk of infection.
- If you are visiting your grandchildren, be extra vigilant about personal hygiene. Avoid contact with children with known infections, such as a cold or the flu; explain that you can become ill very easily, so kissing or holding a child with a known infection is off-limits for you. Wash your hands even more frequently, using paper towels to keep

germs lingering on the family hand towels away from you.

- If someone you intend to visit, including family, is diagnosed with a contagious illness, consider delaying the trip until everyone is well.
- Keep a list in your wallet showing your medical conditions and all medications you take (including over-the-counter medications and supplements you take regularly). If you should become ill while away from home, show the list to the attending physician.

Long-Term Care Facilities

Because of advances in science and technology, we are all living longer lives. While it's not uncommon to live to be 80 or even 90, many aging adults will spend some time in long-term care facilities or nursing homes for either personal or health reasons. These patients are already at increased risk for infection, and the infectious diseases are increasingly resistant to drugs commonly used to treat them.

In a study published in the *Journal of the American Medical Association*, researchers compared healthy nursing home patients with those harboring antibiotic-resistant bacteria. Researchers identified three key reasons for the spread of resistant infections: overuse of antibiotics, low hand washing rates among personnel, and patient transfers between the nursing home and a hospital.

If you or a loved one currently resides in or is considering moving to a long-term care facility, take the steps outlined in the hospitalization section on page 308, plus the tips below, to reduce the risks of getting infected:

- Make sure your immunizations are up-to-date, and consider getting an annual flu shot. In older adults, this vaccine can reduce the severity of influenza and may even prevent it altogether. Each year, the CDC examines epidemiological data to determine which strain of flu will be the most prevalent and develops a new vaccine to fight it. If you are allergic to eggs, specifically ask whether the vaccine is safe for you.

- Ask your doctor about getting a pneumococcal vaccine, which may be underused in nursing homes. (Studies have documented pneumonia outbreaks in nursing homes where fewer than 5 percent of residents had been vaccinated.) This remarkable vaccine can provide immunity against 20 to 30 subtypes of bacteria that commonly cause pneumonia. Some geriatric doctors recommend this vaccine for healthy adults over 65 as well as for younger people at increased risk for infection, such as those with chronic medical problems including liver or heart disease, chronic obstructive pulmonary disease (COPD), kidney failure, diabetes, cancer, and sickle-cell anemia.

Taking Control of Overkill

A resistant bacterial infection could dramatically change your life, but it's important to realize that you have a good deal of control over your health. If you or a loved one has a high Risk Quotient or falls into one of the special categories outlined in this chapter, learn all you can about bacterial resistance. Talk to your doctor about the strategies recommended here, and ask about other preventive measures you can take, depending on your situation. Openly communicate with health care practitioners, friends, teachers, and neighbors about your bacterial concerns.

No matter what your situation, you can improve your well-being and your quality of life. Active participation in your health care, preventive hygiene, and early detection and treatment of bacterial illness are all critical. You can not only improve your own health but also help bring about a healthier future for all of us—a future in which all bacteria are not considered our enemies, and overkill is a thing of the past.

EPILOGUE

A LOOK TO THE FUTURE

This book began with a historical perspective that led up to the present, and it would be unfinished without a glimpse into the future. As a risk analyst, I am familiar not only with predictions of future hazards but also of their importance in helping us imagine and plan for the things to come—for what *might* happen.

Who could have predicted the violent acts of terrorism that occurred in the United States on September 11, 2001, leaving thousands of people dead? What about the subsequent bioterrorism attacks with anthrax? These evil exploits irreversibly changed the lives of millions in our nation and across the globe. They, with the help of a popular book, also woke us up to the clear and present reality that we are vulnerable, both as a nation and as individuals.

The future brings uncertainty, but with it comes tremendous hope. Countless scientific discoveries continue to reveal new ways to battle a variety of deadly germs and once-incurable illnesses. The current revolution in science, particularly such efforts as the human genome project and the technologies emerging from our new understanding of the genetic codes of life, opens the door to rapid diagnostic techniques that may forever alter the way we identify and treat disease.

With each day, we grow closer to the development of medical devices that will quickly identify particular pathogens, telling us whether our symptoms are the result of a bacterial, viral, fungal, or parasitic cause. While medical science is still far away from creating a *Star Trek* "tricorder"—a hand-held device doctors use to scan the body to detect and treat specific ailments—this is a concept that lies within the realm of possibility. Such new technology could not only optimize treatment, but it could prevent the misuse of the tools in our pharmaceutical arsenal by enabling doctors to detect bacterial resistance to specific antibiotics. Another consequence of these medical and technological breakthroughs could be greater awareness of how certain genes lead to increased vulnerability or protection. Perhaps we will soon be able to explore the gene-environment interactions and how they affect the risks of disease.

While the future holds much promise, it also holds some frightening possibilities, including the ongoing threat of terrorism. But planes and bombs are not the only hazards. Just as smallpox once decimated the Native American population, the release today of smallpox—or any other biological weapon—could similarly kill millions of innocent people. Government training exercises documented the enormous potential impact of some scenarios. While some Americans may focus on the small death toll from the anthrax attacks, we should take this as a serious warning signal that we need a comprehensive biodefense system. Instead of hiding in fear, we must recognize and prepare for this potential risk at all levels of government, in health care facilities, and as individuals.

Clear answers to biological threats will depend greatly on the situation, but there *are* steps you can take to protect yourself and your loved ones. First and foremost, be sure your sources of information are credible, such as a government spokesperson or a reliable news agency.

Widespread panic can result from unsubstantiated rumors and misinformation: Shortly following the September 11 attack, there was a run on gas masks, even though experts advised that the masks people were buying were Army surplus and thus outdated and that they would offer little protection in the event of a modern attack. Also consider the following responses if you're concerned about a biological threat:

- Understand that biological weapons generally depend on transmission between people. Unlike physical acts of terrorism (such as plane crashes and bombs) where many people are required to respond by going to help others on the scene, in the case of a biological weapon, the natural tendency to help others could place you at risk. The most appropriate course of action may be to stay home and isolate yourself and your family unless you are properly trained and specifically asked to respond to the biological hazard.
- Prepare your family for periods of isolation. Maintain a stock of several days' worth of bottled water and canned and dried food. This does not mean you should set these supplies aside indefinitely, but use and replace them occasionally so that they remain fresh. For those of you with large pantries full of cans, you're probably already prepared; add an ample supply of bottled water and juices to your pantry too.
- Keep water disinfection tablets, as discussed on page 306, and a well-stocked first aid kit in your home and with you when you travel.
- Make sure you know where to get credible local information about other precautions that may be needed during a crisis. For example, if the biological pathogen is spread via water, then you will need to know whether it's safe to drink water from your tap, to drink it after boiling, to use the water for showering and cleaning, or not to use it at all. If the pathogen is spread in the air, you will need to know how to

deal with this too. Make sure you know when you should go outside, open windows, or even isolate each person in the family. Also ask questions about dealing with the family pets to ensure your safety and theirs.

- Be respectful of others and avoid knowingly exposing others to disease. This means seeking appropriate medical care and isolating yourself, if necessary, to avoid spreading germs to others.

- Report suspicious activities to the proper authorities, such as if you see someone not associated with an establishment putting something into a salad bar or spraying something on others in a crowded room.

- If you become ill after being at a restaurant or other public outing, make sure to write down everything, including the name and number of the place where you ate and all of the places that you have been. Report cases of serious illness to the local public health department and to your physician, even if you don't seek medical care.

- If you suspect a food-borne illness, be sure to report this to the server of the food so that others can also be alerted.

- Keep a copy of your medical history and emergency information up-to-date. Make sure all members of your family receive their recommended immunizations.

- Understand your role in a crisis and follow instructions. As cities develop response strategies, consider innovative opportunities for being part of the response. Get training that you would need to be effective, but stay out of the way if you don't have this training or you're not needed.

We are in a new era, one that unfortunately includes terrorism and biological warfare. But that does not mean we cannot continue to live life to the fullest. It simply means we have to deal with both the known and emerging risks. With increased globalization, we can anticipate an even greater spread of germs and disease between people and nations.

Still, in the Age of Risk Management, we should see not only the risks but also what we can do about them. We must appreciate the power of cooperation and our accomplishments of the past, including global eradication of smallpox and near global eradication of polio and measles. These important examples demonstrate our ability to improve health globally, even as the population of the world continues to grow and place increasing demands on the resources we share. We must also appreciate that by recognizing that there will never be zero risk, we can make choices and take actions that protect health and ensure the highest quality of life. Anything else would be overkill.

REFERENCES

The studies and works referenced in this book are listed below by chapter and page number. Sources that provide a general overview are noted with an asterisk (*). Further, a list of Web sites that provide additional information may be found at www.aorm.com

Introduction

2 Mead, P. S., et al. "Food-Related Illness and Death in the United States." *Emerging Infectious Diseases* 5 (September–October 1999): 607–25.

2 Institute of Medicine. *Antimicrobial Resistance: Issues and Options.* Washington, D.C.: National Academy Press, 1998.

2 *Levy, S. B. *The Antibiotic Paradox: How the Misuse of Antibiotics Destroys Their Curative Powers.* New York: Perseus Books Group, 2001.

2 *Garrett, L. *The Coming Plague: Newly Emerging Diseases in a World Out of Balance.* New York: Farrar, Straus, and Giroux, 1994.

3 Doern, G. V., et al. "Antimicrobial Resistance with *Streptococcus pneumoniae* in the United States, 1997–98." *Emerging Infectious Diseases* 5 (November–December 1999): 121–24.

3 Kronenberger, C. B., et al. "Invasive Penicillin-Resistant Pneumococcal Infections: A Prevalence and Historical Cohort Study." *Emerging Infectious Diseases* 2 (April–June 1996): 121–24.

3 Ohye, R., et al. "Fluoroquinolone Resistance in *Neisseria gonorrhoeae*, Hawaii, 1999, and Decreased Susceptibility to Azithromycin in *N. gonorrhoeae*, Missouri, 1999." *Journal of the American Medical Association* 284 (18 October 2000): 1917–19.

3 Davis, M. A., et al. "Changes in Antimicrobial Resistance among *Salmonella enterica* Serovar Typhimurium Isolates from Humans and Cattle in the Northwestern United States, 1982–1997." *Emerging Infectious Diseases* 5 (November–December 1999): 802–806.

3 Tenover, F. C. "Increasing Resistance to Vancomycin and Other Glycopeptides in *Staphylococcus aureus.*" *Emerging Infectious Diseases* 7 (March–April 2001): 327–32.

3 Lindenmayer, J. M., et al. "Methicillin-Resistant *Staphylococcus aureus* in a High School Wrestling Team and the Surrounding Community." *Archives of Internal Medicine* 158 (27 April 1998): 895–99.

3 Ridzon, R., et al. "Outbreak of Drug-Resistant Tuberculosis with Second-Generation Transmission in a High School in California." *Journal of Pediatrics* 131 (December 1997): 863–68.

3 Blendon, R. J., et al. "Harvard School of Public Health/Robert Wood Johnson Foundation Survey Project on Americans' Response to Biological Terrorism, Tabulation Report, Oct. 24–28, 2001." Media, PA: International Communications Research, 2001.

4 Institute of Medicine. *Antimicrobial Resistance: Issues and Options.* Washington, D.C.: National Academy Press, 1998.

5 Bauchner, H., et al. "Parents, Physicians, and Antibiotic Use." *Pediatrics* 103 (February 1999): 395–401.

5 Mangione-Smith, R., et al. "Parent Expectations for Antibiotics, Physician-Parent Communication, and Satisfaction." *Archives of Pediatrics and Adolescent Medicine* 155 (July 2001): 800–806.

5 Skull, S. A., et al. "Child Care Center Staff Contribute to Physician Visits and Pressure for Antibiotic Prescription." *Archives of Pediatrics and Adolescent Medicine* 154 (February 2000): 180–83.

8 *Meletis, C. D. *Instant Guide to Drug-Herb Interactions*. New York: Dorling Kindersley Publishing, Inc., 2001.

9 Mead, P. S., et al. "Food-Related Illness and Death in the United States." *Emerging Infectious Diseases* 5 (September–October 1999): 607–25.

Chapter 1

12 Crichton, M. *The Andromeda Strain*. New York: Alfred A. Knopf, Inc., 1969.

20 Mead, P. S., et al. "Food-Related Illness and Death in the United States." *Emerging Infectious Diseases* 5 (September–October 1999): 607–25.

29 Rubin, R. J., et al. "The Economic Impact of *Staphylococcus aureus* Infection in New York City Hospitals." *Emerging Infectious Diseases* 5 (January–February 1999): 9–17.

29 Blumberg, H. M., et al. "Rapid Development of Ciprofloxacin Resistance in Methicillin-Susceptible and -Resistant *Staphylococcus aureus*." *Journal of Infectious Diseases* 163 (June 1991): 1279–85.

30 Smith, T. L., et al. "Emergence of Vancomycin Resistance in *Staphylococcus aureus*." *New England Journal of Medicine* 340 (18 February 1999): 493–501.

30 Institute of Medicine. *Antimicrobial Resistance: Issues and Options*. Washington, D.C.: National Academy Press, 1998.

31 Braun, B. L., and J. B. Fowles. "Characteristics and Experiences of Parents and Adults Who Want Antibiotics for Cold Symptoms." *Archives of Family Medicine* 9 (July 2000): 589–95.

32 Nord, C., et al. "Antibiotic Treatment in Patients with Severe Acne Causes Development of Antibiotic Resistance." 101st General Meeting of the American Society for Microbiology, May 2001.

33 Mulvey, M. A., et al. "Establishment of a Persistent *Escherichia coli* Reservoir during the Acute Phase of a Bladder Infection." *Infection and Immunity* 69 (July 2001): 4572–79.

33 Osato, M. S., et al. "Pattern of Primary Resistance of *Helicobacter pylori* to Metronidazole or Clarithromycin in the United States." *Archives of Internal Medicine* 161 (14 May 2001): 1217.

36 Chuanchuen, R., et al. "Cross-Resistance between Triclosan and Antibiotics in *Pseudomonas aeruginosa* Is Mediated by Multidrug Efflux Pumps: Exposure of a Susceptible Mutant Strain to Triclosan Selects nfxB Mutants Overexpressing MexCD-OprJ." *Antimicrobial Agents and Chemotherapy* 45 (February 2001): 428–32.

37 McMurry, L. M., M. Oethinger, and S. B. Levy. "Triclosan Targets Lipid Synthesis." *Nature* 394 (6 August 1998): 531–32.

37 Heath, R. J., and C. O. Rock. "Microbiology: A Triclosan-Resistant Bacterial Enzyme." *Nature* 406 (13 July 2000): 145–46.

37 Riedler, J., et al. "Exposure to Farming in Early Life and Development of Asthma and Allergy: A Cross-Sectional Survey." *The Lancet* 358 (2001): 1129–33.

37 Krämer, U., et al. "Age of Entry to Day Nursery and Allergy in Later Childhood." *The Lancet* 353 (6 February 1999): 450–54.

37 Farooqi, I. S., and J. M. Hopkin. "Early Childhood Infection and Atopic Disorder." *Thorax* 53 (November 1998): 927–32.

37 Alm, J. S., et al. "Atopy in Children of Families with Anthroposophic Lifestyle." *The Lancet* 353 (1 May 1999): 1485–88.

Chapter 2

60 Sanders, S. A., and J. M. Reinisch. "Would You Say You 'Had Sex' If . . . ?" *Journal of the American Medical Association* 281 (20 January 1999): 275–77.

64 *American Society of Microbiology (ASM). "America's Dirty Little Secret—Our Hands." Washington, D.C.: American Society of Microbiology, 2000. Available from www.washup.org/page03.htm.

64 Guinan, M. E., et al. "Who Washes Hands after Using the Bathroom?" *American Journal of Infection Control* 25 (October 1997): 424–25.

64 Harris, A. D., et al. "A Survey on Handwashing and Opinions of Healthcare Workers." *Journal of Hospital Infection* 45 (August 2000): 318–21.

Chapter 3

68 Centers for Disease Control and Prevention (CDC). "About Chronic Disease." Atlanta: Centers for Disease Control and Prevention, 2001. Available from www.cdc.gov/nccdphp/about.htm.

69 Salganik, R. I., 2001. "The Benefits and Hazards of Antioxidants: Controlling Apoptosis and Other Protective Mechanisms in Cancer Patients and the Human Population." *Journal of the American College of Nutrition* 20 (October 2001 Supplement): 464S–75S.

73 Sensakovic, J. W., and L. G. Smith. "Oral Antibiotic Treatment of Infectious Diseases." *Medical Clinics of North America* 85 (January 2001): 115–23.

73 Institute of Medicine. *Antimicrobial Resistance: Issues and Options.* Washington, D.C.: National Academy Press, 1998.

73 Little P., et al. "Clinical and Psychosocial Predictors of Illness Duration from Randomized Controlled Trial of Prescribing Strategies for Sore Throat." *British Medical Journal* 319 (1999): 736–37.

76 American Botanical Council. Available from www.herbalgram.org.

76 Herb Research Foundation. Available from www.herbs.org.

76 National College of Naturopathic Medicine. Available from www.ncnm.edu.

76 The Natural Pharmacist. Available from www.tnp.com.

76 *Balch, P. A., and J. F. Balch. *Prescription for Nutritional Healing.* New York: Avery/The Putnam Publishing Group, 2000.

76 *Blumenthal, M., et al. *The Complete German Commission E Monographs: Therapeutic Guide to Herbal Medicines.* Austin, TX: American Botanical Council, 1999.

76 *Borysenko, J. *Minding the Body, Mending the Mind.* New York: Bantam Books, 1988.

76 *Lininger, S., et al. *The Natural Pharmacy.* Roseville, CA: Prima Publishing, 1999.

76 *Murray, M. T. *Encyclopedia of Nutritional Supplements.* Roseville, CA: Prima Publishing, 1996.

76 *Murray, M. T. *The Healing Power of Herbs.* Roseville, CA: Prima Publishing, 1995.

76 *Robbers, J. E., and V. E. Tyler. *Tyler's Herbs of Choice: The Therapeutic Use of Phytomedicinals.* Binghamton, NY: The Haworth Press, Inc., 1999.

76 *Werbach, M. R. *Nutritional Influences on Illness: A Sourcebook of Clinical Research.* Tarzana, CA: Third Line Press, 1996.

86 Lee, C., and Fan Wan. "Vitamin E Supplementation Improves Cell-Mediated Immunity and Oxidative Stress of Asian Men and Women." *Journal of Nutrition* 130 (December 2000): 2932–37.

86 McGrady A., et al. "The Effects of Biofeedback-Assisted Relaxation on Cell-Mediated Immunity, Cortisol, and White Blood Cell Count in Healthy Adult Subjects." *Journal of Behavioral Medicine* 15 (August 1992): 343–54.

87 Dye, L., et al. "Macronutrients and Mental Performance." *Nutrition* 16 (October 2000): 1021–34.

87 Lyons, P. M., and A. S. Truswell. "Serotonin Precursor Influenced by Type of Carbohydrate Meal in Healthy Adults." *American Journal of Clinical Nutrition* 47 (March 1988): 433–39.

94 Foo, L. Y., et al. "The Structure of Cranberry Proanthocyanidins which Inhibit Adherence of Uropathogenic P-Fimbriated *Escherichia coli* in Vitro." *Phytochemistry* 54 (May 2000): 173–81.

94 Fleet, J. C. "New Support for a Folk Remedy: Cranberry Juice Reduces Bacteriuria and Pyuria in Elderly Women." *Nutrition Reviews* 52 (May 1994): 168–70.

95 Reid, G., et al. "Is There a Role for Lactobacilli in Prevention of Urogenital and Intestinal Infections?" *Clinical Microbiology Reviews* 3 (October 1990): 335–44.

100 Lee, C., and Fan Wan. "Vitamin E Supplementation Improves Cell-Mediated Immunity and Oxidative Stress of Asian Men and Women." *Journal of Nutrition* 130 (December 2000): 2932–37.

103 Maurer, H. R. "Bromelain: Biochemistry, Pharmacology, and Medical Use." *Cellular and Molecular Life Sciences* 58 (August 2001): 1234–45.

104 Bauer, R., et al. "Extract of the *Echinacea purpurea* Herb: An Allopathic Phytoimmunostimulant." In German. *Wiener Medizinische Wochenschrift* 149 (1999): 185–89.

110 *Blumenthal, M., et al. *The Complete German Commission E Monographs: Therapeutic Guide to Herbal Medicines*. Austin, TX: American Botanical Council, 1998.

112 Godfrey, J. C., et al. "Zinc Gluconate and the Common Cold: A Controlled Clinical Study." *Journal of International Medical Research* 20 (June 1992): 234–46.

112 Prasad, A. S., et al. "Duration of Symptoms and Plasma Cytokine Levels in Patients with the Common Cold Treated with Zinc Acetate: A Randomized, Double-Blind, Placebo-Controlled trial." *Annals of Internal Medicine* 133 (15 August 2000): 245–52.

113 Cohen, S., et al. "Psychological Stress and Susceptibility to the Common Cold." *New England Journal of Medicine* 325 (29 August 1991): 606–12.

113 Douglas, R. M., et al. "Vitamin C for Preventing and Treating the Common Cold." *Cochrane Database of Systematic Reviews* 2 (2000): CD000980.

113 Hemila, H. "Vitamin C Supplementation and Common Cold Symptoms: Factors Affecting the Magnitude of the Benefit." *Medical Hypotheses* 52 (February 1999): 171–78.

113 Guinan, M. E., et al. "Who Washes Hands after Using the Bathroom?" *American Journal of Infection Control* 25 (October 1997): 424–25.

125 Capurso, L., et al. "Dietary Fiber in Internal Medicine." In Italian. *Recenti Progressi in Medicina* 87 (July–August 1996): 374–89.

125 Eggenberger, J. C. "Diverticular Disease." *Current Treatment Options in Gastroenterology* 2 (December 1999): 507–16.

131 Zakay-Rones, Z., et al. "Inhibition of Several Strains of Influenza Virus in Vitro and Reduction of Symptoms by an Elderberry Extract (*Sambucus nigra* L.) during an Outbreak of Influenza B Panama." *Journal of Alternative and Complementary Medicine* 1 (Winter 1995): 361–69.

145 Ponikau J. U., et al. "The Diagnosis and Incidence of Allergic Fungal Sinusitis." *Mayo Clinic Proceedings* 74 (September 1999): 877–84.

152 Maurer, H. R. "Bromelain: Biochemistry, Pharmacology, and Medical Use." *Cellular and Molecular Life Sciences* 58 (August 2001): 1234–45.

157 Cheney, G. "Rapid Healing of Peptic Ulcers in Patients Receiving Fresh Cabbage Juice." *California Medicine* 70 (1949): 10–14.

160 Foo, L. Y., et al. "The Structure of Cranberry Proanthocyanidins which Inhibit Adherence of Uropathogenic P-Fimbriated *Escherichia coli* in Vitro." *Phytochemistry* 54 (May 2000): 173–81.

160 Fleet, J. C. "New Support for a Folk Remedy: Cranberry Juice Reduces Bacteriuria and Pyuria in Elderly Women." *Nutrition Reviews* 52 (May 1994): 168–70.

Chapter 4

167 Bauchner, H., et al. "Parents, Physicians, and Antibiotic Use." *Pediatrics* 103 (February 1999): 395–401.

167 Schrag, S. J., et al. "Effect of Short-Course, High-Dose Amoxicillin Therapy on Resistant Pneumococcal Carriage: A Randomized Trial." *Journal of the American Medical Association* 286 (4 July 2001): 49–56.

167 Block, S. L. "Strategies for Dealing with Amoxicillin Failure in Acute Otitis Media." *Archives of Family Medicine* 8 (January/February 1999): 68.

167 Culpepper, L., and J. Froom. "Routine Antimicrobial Treatment of Acute Otitis Media: Is It Necessary?" *Journal of the American Medical Association* 278 (26 November 1997): 1643–45.

167 Finkelstein, J. A., et al. "Antimicrobial Use in Defined Populations of Infants and Young Children. *Archives of Pediatrics and Adolescent Medicine* 154 (April 2000): 395–400.

167 Jacques, L. B., et al. "Antibiotic Prescribing and Respiratory Tract Infections." *Journal of the American Medical Association* 279 (28 January 1998): 271.

167 Skull, S. A., et al. "Child Care Center Staff Contribute to Physician Visits and Pressure for Antibiotic Prescription." *Archives of Pediatrics and Adolescent Medicine* 154 (February 2000): 180–83.

170 Ball, T. M., et al. "Siblings, Day-Care Attendance, and the Risk of Asthma and Wheezing during Childhood." *New England Journal of Medicine* 343 (24 August 2000): 538–43.

170 Krämer, U., et al. "Age of Entry to Day Nursery and Allergy in Later Childhood." *The Lancet* 353 (6 February 1999): 450–54.

170 Farooqi, I. S., and J. M. Hopkin. "Early Childhood Infection and Atopic Disorder." *Thorax* 53 (November 1998): 927–32.

171 Alm, J. S., et al. "Atopy in Children of Families with Anthroposophic Lifestyle." *The Lancet* 353 (1 May 1999): 1485–88.

174 Wong, C. S., et al. "The Risk of the Hemolytic-Uremic Syndrome after Antibiotic Treatment of *Escherichia coli* O157:H7 Infections." *New England Journal of Medicine* 342 (29 June 2000): 1930–36.

181 Hanratty, B., et al. "UK Measles Outbreak in Non-Immune Anthroposophic Communities: The Implications for the Elimination of Measles from Europe." *Epidemiology and Infection* 125 (October 2000): 377–83.

181 Roberts, L., et al. "Effect of Infection Control Measures on the Frequency of Diarrheal Episodes in Child Care: A Randomized, Controlled Trial." *Pediatrics* 105 (April 2000): 743–46.

181 ———. "Effect of Infection Control Measures on the Frequency of Upper Respiratory Infection in Child Care: A Randomized, Controlled Trial." *Pediatrics* 105 (April 2000): 738–42.

181 Carabin, H., et al. "Effectiveness of a Training Program in Reducing Infections in Toddlers Attending Day Care Centers." *Epidemiology* 10 (May 1999): 219–27.

181 Hammond, B., et al. "Effect of Hand Sanitizer Use on Elementary School Absenteeism." *American Journal of Infection Control* 28 (October 2000): 340–46.

183 Rutala, W. A., et al. "Antimicrobial Activity of Home Disinfectants and Natural Products against Potential Human Pathogens." *Infection Control and Hospital Epidemiology* 21 (January 2000): 33–38.

188 Roberts, L., et al. "Effect of Infection Control Measures on the Frequency of Diarrheal Episodes in Child Care: A Randomized, Controlled Trial." *Pediatrics* 105 (April 2000): 743–46.

188 ———. "Effect of Infection Control Measures on the Frequency of Upper Respiratory Infection in Child Care: A Randomized, Controlled Trial." *Pediatrics* 105 (April 2000): 738–42.

195 Magnon, G. J., et al. "Repellency of Two DEET Formulations and Avon Skin-So-Soft Against Biting Midges (Diptera: Ceratopogonidae) in Honduras." *Journal of the American Mosquito Control Association* 7 (March 1991): 80–82.

195 Mafong E. A., and L. A. Kaplan. "Insect repellants: What really works?" *Postgraduate Medicine* 102 (August 1997): 63, 68–69, 74.

195 Peterson, C., et al. "Examination of Two Essential Oils as Mosquito Repellents." Abstract AGRO 73 [453095]. 222nd National Meeting of the American Chemical Society, August 2001.

198 Hashimoto, Y., et al. "Assessment of Magnesium Status in Patients with Bronchial Asthma." *Journal of Asthma* 37 (September 2000): 489–96.

224 Godfrey, J. C., et al. "Zinc Gluconate and the Common Cold: A Controlled Clinical Study." *Journal of International Medical Research* 20 (June 1992): 234–46.

224 Prasad, A. S., et al. "Duration of Symptoms and Plasma Cytokine Levels in Patients with the Common Cold Treated with Zinc Acetate: A Randomized, Double-Blind, Placebo-Controlled trial." *Annals of Internal Medicine* 133 (15 August 2000): 245–52.

224 Rosanowski, F., et al. "Refluxassoziierte Erkankungen im HNO-Bereich." In German. *Laryngorhinootologie* 80 (August 2001): 487–96.

231 Grossan, M. "Irrigation of the Child's Nose: Successful Application of a Dental Pulsating Irrigation Device." *Clinical Pediatrics* 13 (March 1974): 229–31.

Chapter 5

238 Richert, R. J., et al. "Survival and Growth of *E. coli* O157:H7 on Produce." *Journal of Food Protection* 58 (1995 Supplement): 19.

238 Scott, E. "Foodborne Disease and Other Hygiene Issues in the Home." *Journal of Applied Bacteriology* 80 (January 1996): 5.

239 Gerba, C. "You Could Eat Your Dinner Off That . . ." *New Scientist* 158 (13 June 1998): 21.

245 Rutala, W. A., et al. "Antimicrobial Activity of Home Disinfectants and Natural Products against Potential Human Pathogens." *Infection Control and Hospital Epidemiology* 21 (January 2000): 33–38.

247 ———. "Antimicrobial Activity of Home Disinfectants and Natural Products against Potential Human Pathogens." *Infection Control and Hospital Epidemiology* 21 (January 2000): 33–38.

250 Peters, D., et al. "Control of Pathogenic Bacteria on Fresh Produce, a Paper." 83rd Annual Meeting of the International Association of Milk, Food and Environmental Sanitarians, 2 July 1996.

256 Park, P. K., and D. O. Cliver. "Disinfection of Household Cutting Boards with a Microwave Oven." *Journal of Food Protection* 59 (October 1996): 1049–54.

262 Raloff, J. "Sponges and Sinks and Rags, Oh My! Where Microbes Lurk and How to Rout Them." *Science News* 150 (September 1996): 172–73).

Chapter 6

277 Mead, P. S., et al. "Food-Related Illness and Death in the United States." *Emerging Infectious Diseases* 5 (September–October 1999): 607–25.

279 Smith, K. E., et al. "Quinolone-Resistant *Campylobacter jejuni* Infections in Minnesota, 1992–1998." *New England Journal of Medicine* 340 (20 May 1999): 1525–32.

286 *American Society of Microbiology (ASM). "America's Dirty Little Secret—Our Hands." Washington, D.C.: American Society of Microbiology, 2000. Available from www.washup.org/page03.htm.

295 Schwartz, J., R. Levin, and K. Hodge. "Drinking Water Turbidity and Pediatric Hospital Use for Gastrointestinal Illness in Philadelphia." *Epidemiology* 8 (November 1997): 615–20.

Chapter 7

301 Raisler, J., et al. "Breast-Feeding and Infant Illness: A Dose-Response Relationship?" *American Journal of Public Health* 89 (January 1999): 25–30.

304 Ryan, M. A. K., et al. "Handwashing and Respiratory Illness among Young Adults in Military Training." *American Journal of Preventive Medicine* 21 (August 2001): 79–83.

309 Foca, M., et al. "Endemic *Pseudomonas aeruginosa* Infection in a Neonatal Intensive Care Unit." *New England Journal of Medicine* 343 (7 September 2000): 695–700.

309 Harris, A. D., et al. "A Survey on Handwashing and Opinions of Healthcare Workers." *Journal of Hospital Infection* 45 (August 2000): 318–21.

311 Wiener, J., et al. "Multiple Antibiotic-Resistant *Klebsiella* and *Escherichia coli* in Nursing Homes." *Journal of the American Medical Association* 281 (10 February 1999): 517–523.

312 Drinka, P. J. "In Re-Preventing the Spread of Vancomycin-Resistant Enterococci in a Long-Term Care Facility." *Journal of the American Geriatrics Society* 49 (June 2001): 835–37.

Epilogue

313 Miller, J., et al. *Germs: Biological Weapons and America's Secret War.* New York: Simon & Schuster, 2001.

INDEX

Underscored page references indicate boxed text.

A

B

C

D

E

F

H

L

M

N

O

P

Q

R

S

Y

Z